Reversing
Fibromyalgia

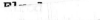

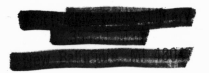

2ND EDITION
REVISED & UPDATED

Reversing Fibromyalgia

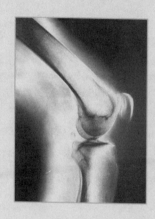

The Whole-Health Approach to Overcoming Fibromyalgia Through Nutrition, Exercise, Supplements and Other Lifestyle Factors

DR. JOE M. ELROD

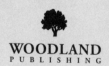

WOODLAND
PUBLISHING

The CIP record for this book is available from the Library of Congress.

For ordering information, contact:
Woodland Publishing, P.O. Box 160, Pleasant Grove, Utah 84062
(800) 777-2665

Note: The information in this book is for educational purposes only and is not recommended as a means of diagnosing or treating an illness. All matters concerning physical and mental health should be supervised by a health practitioner knowledgeable in treating that particular condition. Neither the publisher nor author directly or indirectly dispenses medical advice, nor do they prescribe any remedies or assume any responsibility for those who choose to treat themselves.

ISBN 1-58054-326-X

10 9 8 7 6 5 4 3 2 1

Printed in the United States of America

Please visit our website:
www.woodlandpublishing.com

10/02
D&T
16.95

616.74
LE

Acknowledgments

THE COMPLETION OF this book awakened me to the fact that it is not the end of anything; it is the beginning. A continuation of effort, investigation, persistence and commitment, to pursue answers and hope for those individuals and families who are impacted by this dilemma, as well as other challenging systemic conditions. I wish to recognize all those who have assisted me directly or indirectly in formulating and expressing the research and knowledge shared on the pages of this book.

They include first and foremost my family; my late mother, who was always my biggest fan, gave me life and was always there through the best and worst; my late father, who gave me toughness, determination, and forever pushed me toward excellence; my children and grandchildren, who have, from the first day I witnessed the miracle of the gift of their life, unknowingly inspired me to greater heights; my brother, who has always cared for me, been my mentor and inspiration, and instilled in me a never-say-die attitude when challenged with obstacles.

I also wish to acknowledge my wife, who is my best friend on earth, my soul mate, confidant and life partner. Her confidence and belief in me and all that I do inspires my efforts and creativity. Her love for all living creatures, zest for life, pure heart, spiritual depth, and laughter teach me continuously of all the good things in life and restore my faith in my fellow man.

I express my gratitude to my colleagues, Dr. Bill Hennen and Dr. Cal McCausland, for whom I have great respect as human beings, biochemists, and scientists, and who gave me the great inspiration to write this book. Thanks to my students and patients with whom I have had an association over the years as a university professor, classroom teacher, researcher, health

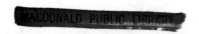

practitioner, and author; they have taught me more than they will ever know.

Special thanks and appreciation goes to my good friend, Mark Victor Hansen, the master motivator and co-author of the remarkable record-setting *Chicken Soup for the Soul* series. Mark endorses this book and inspires me with his dedication to reach and impact millions with his creative works. He accomplishes this through speaking, his books, audios, videos, and his infectious enthusiasm as a remarkable human being.

I also want to thank Annie Kitchens, my all-star computer guru and administrative assistant, who, with great skill and patience, toiled creatively through many late nights and early mornings transforming "Greek" into the beautiful crisp words you are reading this moment. She is a joy to have in our family and on our team.

I want to express appreciation to my editors for their brilliant editing and creative design.

Many thanks to Mark Lisonbee, who originally believed this would be a worthy pursuit to impact millions of individual lives, families, and marriages worldwide.

Finally, I owe a debt of gratitude to my publisher, Calvin Harper, for his dedication, persistence and belief in me and the good cause of this project.

This book, especially the program between its covers, has been a most rewarding enterprise and journey—a journey that will continue on into the undetermined future.

Cervantes said it best: "The road traveled is more rewarding than the end."

Contents

Author's Note

When research for this book began more than ten years ago, very little information on the topic of fibromyalgia existed. When this book was first published just four years ago in 1997, it was only one of a few.

A large number of books have since been published and some outstanding research continues to be done by capable medical scientists in clinics, labs and medical centers around the world. The updated second edition of *Reversing Fibromyalgia* reflects these advances in research and understanding about fibromyalgia's causes and treatment.

How Is This Book Different?

In a recent survey, Barnes&Noble.com listed seventy-seven books with fibromyalgia in the title. Unfortunately, most of these books present protocols that offer only to help manage pain or help one live better with the condition. My book, on the other hand, offers a reversal model with extensive chapters that suggest steps, resources and programs that reverse the condition, not just manage it. Testimonials placed throughout this edition speak to the success of my reversal protocol.

How To Use This Book

I have designed this book so that each section represents a step in the reversal protocol. The first part of this book explains what fibromyalgia is, how to diagnose it, and how to begin to get to where you want to be. The second part outlines nutrition, detoxification programs, nutritional supplements, exercise and stress management tips meant to reverse the condition and restore health.

As you read, you may find that you will eventually need to make several major adjustments in your lifestyle. Although you will need to begin to make some changes in several areas initially, take baby steps at first. For example:

- Adjust your eating patterns gradually.
- Begin to exercise with low impact activities, including easy stretches and low resistance exercises, and progress gradually as your sleep and energy levels return to normal.
- Start a simple regimen of natural supplements gradually moving to a more complete regimen as you progress.
- Adjust your sleep habits and stress management skills gradually as you use the following chapters as your study guide.
- Read this book several times, highlight sections that you really want to emphasize, make notes in it, carry it around and use it consistently. Every time you read or review it you will see something different, mainly because time has passed, progress has been made, and at that point something else applies to you specifically. In other words, become a good student, and it will pay you huge dividends.

Remember that my protocol is based on twenty years of research. As you read this book and attempt to make decisions about this program, you should consider the following facts:

- Fibromyalgia impacts every individual in a different way, and no two people will respond the same way to the treatment regimens outlined in this book.
- This program is very safe and can be very effective. Even if you have severe fibromyalgia, you can still expect to receive dramatic relief; it may just take a bit longer than a person with a less severe form of the syndrome.
- Although this program has not worked 100 percent for all individuals who have tried it, you can fully expect to make progress and even reverse fibromyalgia if you commit fully to this program. Remember, the program in this book is

designed to treat your condition, not simply mask the symptoms to relieve pain temporarily. I have found that many of those who did not find relief with the program did not stick with it consistently. In one particular case, an individual did not begin to see drastic positive results until after almost a year on the program. For some of you, it took a good part of your lifetime to get where you are; therefore, recovery is not an overnight process by any means.

- This program represents a total life management plan and should not be considered only for fibromyalgia, arthritis, migraines or other systemic conditions. This program is designed for every individual who is health conscious and wishes to be proactive in achieving and maintaining health and vitality.

We now know that fibromyalgia can be more than managed—it can be reversed. People simply do not have to accept the bleak prognosis that they will have to live with it the rest of their lives. May the guidelines in this book provide you with the information and impetus to overcome your condition and live a healthier, happier life.

Your Challenge For Renewed Health

How would you like for me to help you regain vital health and self-esteem in just weeks?

What is your dream? Is it to be pain free and energetic once again, to sleep peacefully and wake up refreshed, to reshape your body, to improve the way you feel about yourself so that you can be more successful with your family, your friendships, your business or other endeavors?

Well, what if I told you that I would provide a program for you right now that has been successful for people worldwide, from all walks of life?

Your response to these questions can change your life forever, or keep you where you are—going in the same direction you have been going and getting the same results you have been getting. Now, what if I made a commitment to be your mentor, your "success coach" if you will?

Would you believe that physicians are using this book and my step-by-step program to reverse fibromyalgia, to improve arthritic conditions, to more efficiently manage diabetes, to lower cholesterol, to lower the risk of heart disease, to help avoid osteoporosis, and for healthy weight loss and weight management programs?

If you make a decision to move in a positive direction to change your life, I will teach you how to invest less than 10 percent of the time available to you and make extraordinary changes in your body, your mind, your self-esteem, and success in your life.

I will outline and help you plan every step of the process. I'll help you stay on track, bounce back from setbacks, and in realizing your full potential. My goal is to help you realize your goal of a healthier body, a more powerful mind, a more confident will power, and a higher self-respect. Remember that until we get our bodies in order, it is much more difficult to achieve goals in all other areas.

My program will teach you how to attain (pain free) the strong, healthy body without without spending long, boring hours in a gym and without starving yourself. I will even teach you how to tone your body and lose fat while occasionally enjoying your favorite foods each week.

Imagine waking in the morning, fully rested, full of energy, and truly excited about the person you see in the mirror! Just visualize ten to twenty weeks from now, a new you with energy, health and confidence to go vigorously from early morning to night with the understanding that you can regain control over and accomplish whatever you set your mind to in the world at large.

Well, the good news is, you absolutely can, and it does not matter if you are fourteen or seventy-four years old, male or female, healthy or unhealthy, have fibromyalgia or other systemic conditions. No matter who you are or what the situation, you do have the power to change.

If you want more inspiration, read the success stories placed throughout this book. These people reached out for my assistance, made a commitment and changed their lives. They are living proof that a program of sound nutrition, natural vitamins and herbal supplements, regular reasonable exercise, effective stress coping, and positive thinking can help you change your life and become a new successful, exuberant you.

So, finally, if you will let me help you say yes to life and success, your decision can catapult you toward peace and fulfillment—springboard you toward your full potential and becoming all that you were intended to be.

Yes, you are unique and no one else has your blueprint (or fingerprint). And you—yes, you—were designed to do special things, to make unique contributions, and to positively influence the lives of your loved ones, your fellow men and the world at large. When you are ready, turn the next page and begin your venture to health, vitality, success and a higher quality of life.

1

What Is Fibromyalgia?

"We first make our habits, and then our habits make us."
— JOHN DRYDEN

What is fibromyalgia? It sounds like a simple question, but scientists have been debating the answer for decades. Although we learn more about fibromyalgia syndrome each year, most doctors will tell you that explaining what fibromyalgia *is not* is sometimes easier than defining what it is—which may explain why it takes as long as five (or more) years after the onset of the disease for it to be accurately identified.

In fact, medical tests done to determine whether a person has fibromyalgia are often necessary to *exclude* other conditions rather than positively establish fibromyalgia as the cause of symptoms. This is because many of its symptoms can point to a number of health problems besides fibromyalgia. As a result, defining and diagnosing fibromyalgia continues to be problematic, and some doctors still do not accept its validity. Critics of fibromyalgia claim that it is just an umbrella term for a number of conditions, but as research continues to be published on the subject, more and more experts are convinced of its existence (White, 2001).

In the mainstream medical community, fibromyalgia is considered an incurable syndrome characterized by generalized musculoskeletal pain, stiffness and chronic aching, but many other seemingly unrelated symptoms are also associated with the syndrome. One identifying characteristic of fibromyalgia is the existence of reproducible tenderness on palpation (a medical term for touching) of specific anatomical sites referred to as *tender points,* which will be discussed in more detail later in this chapter.

The name "fibromyalgia" has largely replaced the earlier term "fibrositis," once used to describe the syndrome. "Itis" means inflammation and earlier research described fibromyalgia syndrome as inflammation in muscles, but during the past fifty years research has all but proven that inflammation is not a significant part of fibromyalgia. The term "fibromyalgia" is considered more accurate because it means *pain* in the muscles and the fibrous connective tissues.

Fibromyalgia is not Arthritis

Some fibromyalgia patients feel pain that is focused in their joints—similar to arthritis—but extensive studies have shown that fibromyalgia patients do not have arthritis. In fact, fibromyalgia pain is not in the joints at all, but in the muscles and ligaments surrounding the joints. Fibromyalgia is really a form of muscular or "soft tissue" rheumatism, rather than arthritis of the joints. The word "rheumatism" refers to the pain or inflammation and stiffness of the joints, muscles or fibrous tissue. Since fibromyalgia syndrome is a *soft tissue* rheumatism, it mainly affects the muscles and their attachments to bones, especially the areas of muscle/tendon junctions (Bennett, 1989).

Why Is Fibromyalgia a "Syndrome"?

Fibromyalgia is referred to as a "syndrome" because it is a set of signs (what the physician finds during an exam) and symptoms (what a patient reports to their doctor during an exam) that occur together. Although some health experts believe that the lack of one identifiable cause raises doubts about the existence of fibromyalgia, many others believe that trying to find only one cause for fibromyalgia is the wrong approach. Instead, each fibromyalgia case should be seen as a unique combination of factors that cause the syndrome. Although general symptoms and causal factors may be somewhat consistent among fibromyalgia patients, specific combinations and factors will vary from person to person, as should treatment.

A Short History of Fibromyalgia

No one knows exactly how long fibromyalgia has been around, but "tender points" were first identified by a Scottish researcher in the early 1800s. Throughout that century, various names and symptoms were associated with tender point pain, but it wasn't until the start of the twentieth century that doctors agreed on the term "fibrositis." From that point until the late 80s, there was a large amount of disagreement over the existence, causes and symptoms of the syndrome. However, in 1987, fibromyalgia was finally recognized by the American Medical Association (AMA) as legitimate because of a landmark *JAMA* study published that year on the symptoms of fibromyalgia. Not long after the study, in 1993, fibromyalgia was also recognized by the World Health Organization (WHO). The disease was described not as a psychologically driven illness, as it had been previously categorized, but as a painful muscle syndrome that caused widespread fatigue, sleep disorders, depression, and anxiety. Since then, research funding for the study of fibromyalgia has more than tripled, and new information about fibromyalgia is discovered and published each year.

The Symptoms of Fibromyalgia

I mentioned earlier that a number of symptoms are associated with fibromyalgia, some that are directly related to pain in the muscles and connective tissues and some which are not. Below is a short list of some of the more common and accepted symptoms associated with the syndrome:

- anxiety and/or panic attacks
- cardiovascular problems (dizziness, palpitations)
- chronic fatigue and low energy
- chronic, widespread aches and pains
- depression
- gastrointestinal disturbances/irritable bowel syndrome
- intolerance to cold temperatures
- irritable bladder syndrome
- memory and concentration problems, called "fibro fog"
- neck and back pain
- pelvic pain in women (painful menstruation) and/or PMS
- poor circulation (cold hands and feet)
- sleep disturbances and/or restless leg syndrome
- stiffness (especially in the morning) and/or muscle twitching
- subjective soft tissue swelling or paresthesia in hands, arms, feet or legs
- tenderness of at least eleven of eighteen specific anatomical sites (see figure 2 in Chapter 2)
- tension headaches and/or migraines

Of course, there are many other symptoms associated with fibromyalgia. A partial list of these lesser known or less accepted symptoms includes acid reflux and/or trouble swallowing; dry mouth, nose and eyes; hearing, visual or respiratory difficulties; allergies and environmental sensitivities; costochondritis (chest pain in the muscles that can feel like heart pain); vertigo; skin sensitivities; and impaired coordination.

"I Ache All Over"

Most patients with fibromyalgia syndrome state that they literally "ache all over." They describe their muscles as feeling as if they have been pulled, torn or overworked—sometimes twitching and other times burning. The severity of this and other symptoms will fluctuate tremendously from one person to the next. Fibromyalgia syndrome sometimes resembles a post-viral state, which is one of the reasons some experts in the field believe that fibromyalgia syndrome and chronic fatigue syndrome might share etiologies or origins, especially abnormalities in the stress-response system. But current research is uncovering dissimilarities between the two despite overlaps (Naschitz, 2001 and Buskila, 2001) that I will elaborate on later in the chapter.

But as with chronic fatigue syndrome, family, friends and work associates of patients with fibromyalgia very often have a difficult time understanding the condition, especially the pain, because blood tests and x-rays reveal no physical evidence. I suggest that they might think back to the last time they had the flu, when every muscle in the body ached and they felt totally drained of energy. This might help them understand what fibromyalgia feels like.

What About the Pain?

The pain associated with fibromyalgia syndrome is the most prominent symptom of the condition. Patients describe the pain as deep, burning, throbbing and stabbing. The pain is generally felt throughout the body, although it starts in one region such as the neck and shoulders, and then seems to spread over time to other parts of the body. The pain will often vary, depending on the time of day, activity level, the weather, sleep patterns, and interruptions in lifestyle. Most fibromyalgia patients report that some degree of pain is consistently present.

Most often the pain and stiffness are worse in the early morning and in muscles that are used repetitively. In many cases physicians are not familiar with evaluation of the tender points, but rheumatologists (specialists in arthritis and rheumatism) will usually know better when and how to perform the examination to diagnose fibromyalgia syndrome.

Though there appears to be no specific diagnostic test available, recent research suggests that people with fibromyalgia are physiologically different. Dr. Laurence Bradley, professor of medicine at the Division of Clinical Immunology and Rheumatology at the University of Alabama in Birmingham, is leading an investigation into fibromyalgia physiology. The team discovered that the cerebral spinal fluid in those with fibromyalgia contains more substance P, a neuropeptide which serves as a peripheral pain neurotransmitter (carries pain signals). High levels of substance P mean that more pain is perceived by the sufferer. Dr. Bradley says, "It's almost like those with fibromyalgia have a pain filter that's not working well."

Furthermore, according to a November 1998 issue of *Pain*, cerebrospinal levels of substance P were higher than normal in tested fibromyalgia patients, but normal in subjects diagnosed with chronic fatigue syndrome. Nevertheless, the exact triggers for abnormal pain sensitivities and disrupted sleeping patterns in fibromyalgics are still being debated; however, the more prominent theory appears to be severe, long-term stress coupled with emotionally traumatic experiences (Russell, 1996). Crofford (1994) and Moldofsky (1995) have identified similar neuroendocrine abnormalities in other studies that continue to form the basis of the causes of fibromyalgia.

It has also been suggested that fibromyalgia pain is related to microtrauma in deconditioned muscles, and that the right kind of exercise is beneficial for reconditioning these muscles (Bennett, 1989). The Body Advantage exercise system was developed to provide the "right kind" of low impact exercise to help promote healing. (Refer to the Resource Guide for more information.) The tender areas of fibromyalgia, or trigger points, are similar in location to sore and tender areas in other common muscle and bone pain disorders such as tennis elbow and trochanteric bursitis (inflammation of the outer side of the hip). However, those with fibromyalgia very often are not aware of the exact location or even the presence of many of the trigger points until they are specifically examined by a health professional or physician.

The Role of Digestion

Some statistics show that nearly 70 percent of fibromyalgics also suffer from chronic digestive problems. The links between gastrointestinal disturbances and fibromyalgia aren't really that surprising. Links between irritable bowel and depression have already been established. Stress, nutrient deficiencies, food and chemical sensitivities, microbe infections, NSAIDS like aspirin, and anxiety can all trigger digestive problems, and many of these factors also contribute to the genesis or continuation of fibromyalgia in some people. Irritable bowel may explain the fatigue and nutrient malabsorption felt by some fibromyalgics, and the eneroviruses that are currently being linked to the syndrome are often found in the gastrointestinal tract. However, according to a recent study out of Norway, irritable bowel does not seem to be linked to the chronic, widespread pain associated with fibromyalgia (Palm, 2001).

Irritable bowel syndrome's links to other fibromyalgia symptoms remain largely untested. But according to the *Annals of Internal Medicine*, "overlap between unexplained clinical conditions [like fibromyalgia, tension headaches, cystitis and irritable bowel] are substantial" (Aaron, 2001). The factors connecting many unexplained chronic conditions remain unknown in many cases, but because digestion may contribute to fibromyalgia flare-ups to such a large degree, proper diet and nutritional supplementation are essential to the sufferer. The importance of nutrition is discussed in more detail in Chapter 6.

Fatigue and Sleep Disorders

The fatigue associated with fibromyalgia has been described as *brain fatigue* in which people feel totally drained of energy. Fatigue can be mild in some and incapacitating in others. Ninety percent of those with fibromyalgia describe their fatigue as moderate or severe, similar to the exhaustion experienced with the flu. Very often, the fatigue is more problematic than the pain. Many patients state that they feel as if their arms are tied to concrete blocks, and they have great difficulty concentrating.

Furthermore, most will generally have difficulty sleeping and will wake up feeling very tired. Sleeping disorders associated with fibromyalgia are probably one of the more devastating symptoms of the syndrome. During sleep we usually have periods when we stop moving and go into a deep, very restful, recharging sleep (also called level 4 sleep), but scientific studies indicate that most people with fibromyalgia have an abnormal sleep pattern marked by interruptions in their deep sleep. In one study done in a sleep lab, researchers found that those with fibromyalgia could fall asleep without much difficulty at all. However, their deep sleep was constantly interrupted by bursts of awake-like brain activity. This fact coincides with the fact that low levels of growth hormone, important in maintaining good muscles and other soft tissue health, have been found in people with fibromyalgia. This hormone is produced almost exclusively in deep sleep, and its production is increased by exercise.

Unfortunately, in fibromyalgia, the muscle and connective tissue pain makes it impossible to lie in one position for an extended period of time. As a result, the patient is continually brought back into light sleep. Fibromyalgia patients simply do not experience the deep stages of sleep that allow for complete rest. Even when they sleep for eight hours a night, they may awaken tired each morning (May, 1993).

Physicians typically do not have to order expensive sleep lab tests to determine if someone suffers with disturbed sleep. If the individual wakes up feeling as though they have been awake all night, doctors refer to this as "unrefreshed sleep," and it is reasonable for a physician or a health professional to assume or to classify this as a sleeping disorder.

Many fibromyalgia sufferers are diagnosed with an associated deep sleep disorder called *alpha-EEG anomaly*. (Most people diagnosed with chronic fatigue syndrome have the same alpha-EEG sleep pattern.) Also, some fibromyalgia patients have been found to have other sleep disorders, such as sleep apnea (temporary cessation of breathing during sleep), nocturnal myoclonus (nighttime jerking of the arms and legs), restless leg syndrome, and bruxism (unconscious teeth grinding). Furthermore, it has been determined that the sleep pattern for clinically depressed patients is distinctly different from that found in fibromyalgics or those with chronic fatigue syndrome (Moldofsky, 1975).

Fibromyalgia and the Brain

As mentioned, depression, anxiety and mental fogginess are all associated with fibromyalgia syndrome. And along with pain and sleep disorders, these symptoms often interfere the most with normal activities for fibromyalgics. In fact, antidepressants are one of the most commonly prescribed drugs for fibromyalgia, and depression and anxiety may also trigger the onset of fibromyalgia as well as flare-ups. I will discuss the links between fibromyalgia and various neurotransmitters later in this chapter.

Who Is Affected?

Experts estimate that six to ten million Americans suffer from fibromyalgia, but I believe the actual figure is much higher. It is seen in all age groups from young children to the elder-

"My body—and my life—were a wreck"

At age fourteen in my homeland of Russia, I was an Olympic potential cross-country skier. Because of a devastating home situation, I began to self-destruct on drugs. By age seventeen, I was diagnosed with mononucleosis. At age twenty-two, I was diagnosed with chronic fibromyalgia. My body—and my life—were a wreck.

Because of Dr. Elrod's book, Reversing Fibromyalgia, and the breakthrough reversal process of the HOPE Medical Clinic, I now have my life back . . . pain free! I am director of my husband's company; I home school my young son and am taking night classes for an advanced degree.

This program has performed a miracle in my life and given me hope when I had been told there was none!

Ekaterina A.
Ottawa, Canada

ly, although for most patients, the problem begins in their twenties or thirties. Fibromyalgia strikes women more than men—in a ratio of nine to one (Yunus, 2001). But although 90 percent of diagnosed fibromyalgics are said to be women (Anderberg, 2000), according to Dr. Milton Hammerly in his book, *Fibromyalgia: How to Combine the Best of Traditional and Alternative Therapies* (2000), this statistic may be misleading since many men with fibromyalgia may not seek treatment. Women, however, do seem to experience more symptoms than men and reportedly have more fatigue, more widespread pain and more instances of irritable bowel syndrome than men, according to a recent study in *Current Rheumatology Reports* (Yunus, 2001).

Fibromyalgia is also more common in middle-aged women between the ages of thirty and fifty years, but the numbers of younger people with fibromyalgia is growing. In fact, I personally have worked with a nine-year-old girl in Ontario, Canada.

Fibromyalgia in children is referred to as "juvenile primary fibromyalgia syndrome" or JPFS and was discovered in the mid-eighties. In children, fibromyalgia affects more boys than girls.

Fibromyalgia affects approximately 2 to 4 percent of people in industrialized societies (Littlejohn, 2001), and is one of the three most common adult rheumatic diagnoses today (Offenbaecher, 1998). Moreover, it is estimated that only half of those people with fibromyalgia even know they have it because many people ignore symptoms until they are very serious. Also, many doctors misdiagnose fibromyalgia. In fact, experts estimate that it takes approximately *four to five years* from the onset of symptoms in a person until it is recognized.

Is There a Fibromyalgia Personality?

Although there is no scientific research on a possible "fibromyalgia personality," Dr. Mark J. Pellegrino, author of *Inside Fibromyalgia* (2001) and a fibromyalgia survivor, believes that certain character traits may predispose individuals to the illness. Using his experience in the field, he identifies those who are driven, anxious, compulsive, overachievers, organized, perfectionists and "time-oriented" as those most at risk for fibromyalgia. All of these traits are considered fibromyalgia risk factors because they can lead to chronic stress and exhaustion if nothing is done to mitigate their effects.

What Causes Fibromyalgia?

Although the causes of fibromyalgia syndrome remain unsubstantiated or debated, current fibromyalgia researchers have uncovered a number of clues to what triggers fibromyalgia or predisposes someone to develop it. The following list of events and conditions (along with those listed in Figure 1) represent my theory of contributing factors to the onset of fibromyalgia taken from more than ten years of hands-on research. You will probably recognize some causes are also listed as fibromyalgia symptoms earlier in this chapter:

- stress and/or depression
- traumatic emotional/physical experience (i.e. accident, divorce, illness, abuse, etc.)
- accumulation of toxins from refined foods, air, water
- biological disruption of energy production
- chronic fatigue
- disruption of sleep cycle (inability to enjoy prolonged sleep)
- a family history of fibromyalgia, especially in one or both parents
- hypersensitivity (the sensations of pain and other stimuli are amplified by the body)
- overwhelmed or impaired immune system (i.e. low or impaired natural killer cell function)
- prolonged infection or illness
- low levels of growth hormone
- neurotransmitter and nervous system dysfunctions
- nutrient and oxygen deficiencies (i.e. magnesium, selenium, phosphates, substrates)
- poor diet and/or lack of exercise

Close to one hundred percent of the fibromyalgia victims I have personally worked with have experienced a long period of extreme stress or emotional trauma—whether it be an automobile accident, divorce, a long illness, growing up in a dysfunctional family, experiencing abuse as a child or some other type of trauma. Many experts believe that these "triggering events" probably do not cause fibromyalgia but rather *awaken or provoke an underlying physiological abnormality.*

A physical or emotional trauma can precipitate fibromyalgia in a number of ways. For example, a physical trauma such as having an infection or flu can lead to certain hormonal or chemical changes that promote pain and disturbed sleep. Also,

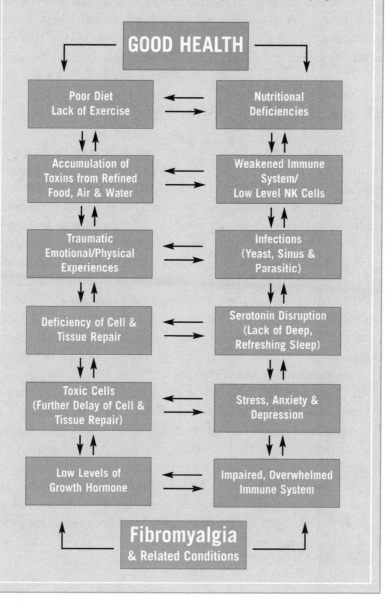

Figure 1. The causes of fibromyalgia

This figure illustrates the "vicious cycle" of events and factors that can contribute to the onset and progression of fibromyalgia.

GOOD HEALTH

Poor Diet
Lack of Exercise

Nutritional
Deficiencies

Accumulation of
Toxins from Refined
Food, Air & Water

Weakened Immune
System/
Low Level NK Cells

Traumatic
Emotional/Physical
Experiences

Infections
(Yeast, Sinus &
Parasitic)

Deficiency of Cell &
Tissue Repair

Serotonin Disruption
(Lack of Deep,
Refreshing Sleep)

Toxic Cells
(Further Delay of Cell &
Tissue Repair)

Stress, Anxiety &
Depression

Low Levels of
Growth Hormone

Impaired, Overwhelmed
Immune System

Fibromyalgia
& Related Conditions

those with fibromyalgia may become inactive because of chronic pain, and they feel anxious about their health, which further aggravates the disorder. In fact, recent studies have shown that in fibromyalgia sufferers' muscles are especially vulnerable to decreased circulation and minor injury. In the following sections, I will discuss links between the physical and psychological triggers listed on the previous page, and theories about how they may precipitate fibromyalgia symptoms.

Suspected Culprits: Stress and Trauma

One theory currently being evaluated as a possible cause of fibromyalgia is the body's response to stress and trauma. Researchers are trying to determine if the autonomic nervous system (which governs involuntary actions) works properly under such conditions. Long periods of undue stress and emotional disruption appear to be the underlying cause of energy compound deficiencies by interrupting the natural physiological process of ATP (energy) production. Disruptions in energy production are also linked to nutrient deficiencies that can be caused by poor diet or digestive malabsorption of needed nutrients. Prolonged stress and trauma, when combined with a poor diet, lack of exercise and certain biological dysfunctions may lead to the onset of fibromyalgia.

In fact, in a recent study published in *Current Rheumatology Reports*, researchers state that fibromyalgia is linked to increased rates of psychiatric disorders like depressive anxiety, and that depression, distress and other psychological factors are linked to "the onset and persistence of fibromyalgia symptoms." They conclude that while the exact cause of fibromyalgia is unclear, sufferers do demonstrate an "altered stress system responsiveness" linked to abnormalities and dysfunctions in the hypothalamus, pituitary and adrenal glands (McBeth, 2001).

The Role of Abuse in Fibromyalgia

In a 2001 issue of *Psychosomatics*, researchers discovered higher incidences of victimization (i.e. emotional and physical abuse) among fibromyalgia (FM) and chronic fatigue (CFS) sufferers than in individuals with rheumatoid arthritis (RA) and multiple sclerosis (MS). CFS and FM patients were more likely to have experienced emotional abuse and neglect and/or physical abuse, particularly lifelong victimization by parents and/or their partners. These findings support the belief that chronic stress plays a pivotal role in the development of chronic fatigue and fibromyalgia syndromes (Van Houdenhove, 2001).

Is Fibromyalgia in the Genes?

Looking back at the list of biological triggers—hormone imbalances, neurotransmitter and immune system dysfunctions, etc., it is easy to see how fibromyalgia could be hereditary, at least to a degree. In fact, some researchers believe that family history can play a role in who gets fibromyalgia, especially if one or more parents have it. And although no research to date has identified a "fibromyalgia gene" to legitimize this claim, research has shown that other symptoms associated with fibromyalgia can be genetic—depression, anxiety, eating disorders.

Hereditary depression has been of particular interest to researchers. One recent study on depression and fibromyalgia found that 23 percent of fibromyalgia sufferers surveyed had a family history of depression, 46 percent had a family history of fibromyalgia and 46 percent had been diagnosed with depression at least once in the past (Offenbaecher, 1998). Another study (Ackenheil, 1998) found that the serotonin transporter promoter gene associated with anxiety and fibromyalgia may provide an example of genetic transmission—genes that can be passed on from parent to child.

Furthermore, a 1999 study found that fibromyalgia patients were not only more likely to have a particular serotonin transporter genotype implicated in altered serotonin metabolism, but also fibromyalgics with this genotype were more prone to depression than healthy control subjects (Offenbaecher). Also, an earlier study links not only hereditary depression to fibromyalgia, but also a history of alcoholism in first degree relatives (Katz, 1996).

The Depression Link to Fibromyalgia

Depression is cited by fibromyalgia experts as both a symptom of the illness and a possible cause or trigger of it. In fact, major depression and fibromyalgia share many of the same symptoms. In *Solving the Depression Puzzle* (2001), Rita Elkins, M.H., lists fibromyalgia as an illness that impacts brain chemistry and worsens depression. Although all of the connections between fibromyalgia and depression are not known or fully understood, researchers are beginning to understand how certain neurotransmitters involved in mood are also linked to the pain and fatigue felt in fibromyalgia patients. For instance, serotonin, a neurochemical that is often studied in association with depression and anxiety, is also connected to muscle and immune functions, pain sensation, and sleep (Dauvilliers, 2001 and Hammerly, 2000).

Some studies have shown that fibromyalgia sufferers tend to be severely deficient in serotonin or suffer from altered serotonin metabolism (Offenbaecher, 1999). For example, a recent study in the *Journal of Orofacial Pain* found that fibromyalgia patients showed much lower serum serotonin levels than patients with rheumatoid arthritis and scored higher on the Spielberger State and Trait Anxiety Inventory (STAI) scale. They also scored higher on tender point tests of orofacial (mouth and face) pain and had a significantly lower pressure pain threshold (or PPT) than healthy individuals tested. They concluded that serotonin imbalances are "associated with pain and discomfort and increased anxiety in fibromyalgia" (Ernberg, 2000).

But some researchers still resist the theory of serotonin deficiencies. A 2001 study in *Rheumatology* does not deny the connection, but they conclude that their research does not confirm the connection either (Legangneux). Nevertheless, numerous studies—like a 2000 study in the *Journal of General Internal Medicine*—have found that serotonin-manipulating antidepressants can be effective in fibromyalgia treatment, which implies that a connection between serotonin and the syndrome must exist.

Moreover, two other neurotransmitters, epinephrine and norepinephrine, that help the body handle stress by regulating heart rate, blood pressure and various immune cells, are also linked to depression. Chronic stress may result in abnormal release of these chemicals in the body, possibly leading to altered nervous system (and immune system) responses and ultimately, fibromyalgia (Elkins, 2001 and Elenkov, 2000).

Substance P and Fibromyalgia Pain

Another neurotransmitter mentioned earlier in the chapter that has been receiving plenty of attention in fibromyalgia research is substance P, the hormone that carries pain signals. Substance P was discovered in the 1930s and has been implicated in such health problems as asthma, chronic bronchitis, cystitis, inflammatory bowel disease, migraines, depression, pain, seizures and chronic inflammatory conditions (Harrison, 2001).

Substance P levels are sometimes *three times higher than normal* in fibromyalgia patients (Hammerly, 2000), and it is believed that the abnormal levels of substance P may explain feelings of generalized pain experienced by sufferers. In fact, serotonin regulates the levels of substance P in the body, so serotonin deficiencies may be responsible for above average amounts of substance P in fibromyalgia victims.

Substance P irregularities may explain one theory of the causes of fibromyalgia. Some doctors believe that fibromyalgia pain is caused by hypersensitivity in certain people. Because of chronic overstimulation, the brain may exaggerate some pain responses and interpret other types of stimulation as pain that are not, perhaps leading to chronic, widespread pain characteristic of fibromyalgia (Aaron, 2001 and De Stefano, 2000).

In fact, new research out of the University of Florida has uncovered another possible explanation for the widespread and tender point pain associated with fibromyalgia. The head researcher, rheumatologist Roland Staud, M.D., believes that the spinal cord of a fibromyalgia sufferer is "sensitized," meaning it can detect very small changes and interprets them as painful, where a normal person would not. He explains that the spinal cord interprets signals it gets from neurotransmitters, and if the spinal cord is damaged by injury or infection in people with an inherited susceptibility, chronic stress or fatigue, this may trigger abnormal sensitivities in the spinal cord that lead to fibromyalgia pain (Remington, 2001).

Neurotransmitters and Muscles

The nervous system not only influences mood and pain responses, but also how our muscles work because they are the messengers between our muscles and the nervous system. If sensory information from these transmitters is faulty, the muscles must do all the work of coordinating and contracting on their own. This dysfunction may, for example, cause muscles to contract more than necessary. Some researchers hypothesize that the muscles in fibromyalgia victims are overworked because of dysfunctional communication between these muscles and the nervous system, which may lead to the pain and fatigue characteristic of the illness. The reasons for these faulty communications are unknown, but chronic stress may be a factor. Other muscle abnormalities may be related to dysfunctional energy production, problems within the muscle fibers and in muscle mitochondria, or endocrine factors (Park, 2000 and Hammerly, 2000).

The Hormone Connection

Chronic stress and fatigue also influence a number of hormones that are currently being studied as possible culprits of fibromyalgia. For instance, cortisol is a stress hormone linked to obesity, diabetes and depression, but recent research also connects it to fibromyalgia symptoms. In a 2000 issue of *Psychoneuroendocrinology*, a phenomenon called "hypocortisolism" (deficient cortisol activity) is linked to stress-related disorders like chronic fatigue, fibromyalgia and rheumatoid arthritis. Previous research only linked low cortisol to posttraumatic stress disorder and other trauma-related events. Researchers in the study believe that "persistent lack of cortisol availability in traumatized or chronically stressed individuals may promote an increased vulnerability for the development of stress-related bodily disorders" (Heim, 2000).

Cortisol activity may also affect estrogen levels in women, according to scientific research. In *Solving the Depression Puzzle* (2001), Elkins mentions a possible link between estrogen and fibromyalgia. Although the specific nature of the connection is not entirely known, changes in estrogen can interfere with serotonin production. Earlier, I mentioned the established relationship between serotonin and fibromyalgia symptoms. If estrogen influences serotonin production, then it is safe to assume that estrogen imbalances in women may also be a factor in fibromyalgia.

In fact, many women with fibromyalgia complain of worsened fibromyalgia symptoms around their periods, and fibromyalgia has also been linked to menopausal problems. Some experts believe that low estrogen supplies (or inefficient use of estrogen in the body) are to blame and that natural hormone replacement therapy may alleviate symptoms of pain and fatigue (Pellegrino, 2001).

Estrogen imbalances can also affect the thyroid gland and the thyrotropin-releasing hormone (TRH), which regulates the thyroid—also implicated in the development of fibromyalgia symptoms, particularly fatigue. TRH stimulates the pituitary gland to produce thyroid stimulating hormones (TSH), which in turn stimulates thyroid production of thyroxin. This is critical simply because thyroxin regulates metabolic rate. Thyroxin irregularities may explain some symptoms of fibromyalgia.

DHEA and Depression

Dehydroepiandrosterone (DHEA), an adrenal gland hormone linked to depression and fatigue (Elkins, 2001), is also found in lower levels in fibromyalgia patients, and a 1994 study suggested that there may be a connection between low DHEA levels and the development of fibromyalgia symptoms (Nilsson). However, a later study published in an issue *Pain* determined that DHEA may be related more to age and body mass index (BMI) than fibromyalgia pain (Dessein, 1999). Nevertheless, many doctors do recommend that fibromyalgia patients get their DHEA levels tested. DHEA supplementation has been linked to increased cancer risk if not used with care, but it has been shown to relieve fibromyalgia symptoms of fatigue, foggy thinking and sleep disorders in some patients (Hammerly, 2000).

Growth Hormones and Fibromyalgia

Another hormone that has received a lot of scientific attention in connection with fibromyalgia is growth hormone. Earlier I mentioned that growth hormone (GH) is almost exclusively produced during deep sleep, which many fibromyalgia patients do not get. GH production is also increased by exercising—another thing many fibromyalgia patients do not get enough of.

Growth hormones are produced by the pituitary gland and are important in metabolism, particularly fat burning and muscle building. In fact, growth hormones break down into a number of particles in the bloodstream, such as insulin-like growth factor I (IGF-I), which monitors growth factor activity. IGF-I levels are often low in fibromyalgia patients, and this deficiency is linked to symptoms of fatigue as well as cold hands and feet (Pellegrino, 2001). Later in the book, I will discuss exercising techniques and supplements designed to stimulate GH production.

However, the results of one recent study showed *no differences* in IGF-I levels between healthy women and women with fibromyalgia even though healthy women showed more growth hormone production during sleep than their fibromyalgia counterparts (Landis, 2001). Despite links between decreased GH production and disorders like fibromyalgia and chronic fatigue, researchers are still not sure if impaired growth hormone secretion is a cause or effect of either condition.

Fibromyalgia and the Immune System

The connection between fibromyalgia symptoms and growth hormones may not be understood, but the syndrome's connection to the immune system is undeniable, especially since research is continuing to establish fibromyalgia as a stress-related disorder. The body's stress responses often suppress immune function, and many of the hormones and neurotransmitters mentioned so far influence immunity (or the reverse).

The body is equipped to handle short-term stress, but chronic stress puts a lot of strain on body systems and their functions. In fact, recent findings have already surfaced linking long-term stress to heart attacks, obesity and diabetes. Also, research on the relationship between immune function and fibromyalgia has uncovered quite a few findings. For instance, natural killer or NK cells, that fight bacteria and other invaders, are less active in fibromyalgia sufferers, and often levels of cytokines, another type of immune cell, are either elevated or deficient in individuals with fibromyalgia (Hammerly, 2000 and Wallace, 2001). This may help explain why fibromyalgia victims are sometimes prone to infections. Depression has also been linked to impaired immune function (Elkins, 2001), and the combined effect of depression and stress may trigger fibromyalgia symptoms by impairing immune function.

Another point of interest to mention when talking about the immune system and infection is the presence of mycoplasmal blood infections in fibromyalgia patients. These parasites fall somewhere between viruses and bacteria, and are present in more than 60 percent of fibromyalgia and chronic fatigue patients. These organisms may eventually reveal more about the causes of fibromyalgia symptoms (Nasralla, 1999).

Individuals with fibromyalgia are also more likely to have certain viral antibodies, according to a 2001 issue of the *Journal of Rheumatology*. Researchers tested fibromyalgia patients for various antibodies and found that half of acute onset patients tested positive for an antibody that fights eneroviruses, typically found in the gastrointestinal tract and associated with meningitis, respiratory illnesses and neurological disorders. They believe that these findings may provide clues about the syndrome's causes and immune response in sufferers (Wittrup). Antibodies against serotonin and thromboplastin are also associated with fibromyalgia, but the significance of these findings is still unknown (Werle, 2001).

The Role of Exercise and Diet

A healthy diet and regular exercise are often championed as the best ways to boost immune function and overall health. Unfortunately, for many fibromyalgia sufferers, these two essential ingredients in disease management are often neglected. Even active individuals who understand the benefits of eating right and exercising may have difficulty following through because of fibromyalgia fatigue, depression and pain.

Although many fibromyalgia patients are aware of pain when they are resting, it is most noticeable when they use their muscles, particularly when exercising. Their discomfort can be so severe it may significantly limit their ability to lead a full life. At times, patients find themselves unable to work or even performing everyday tasks. As a consequence of muscle pain, many fibromyalgia patients severely limit their activities and exercise. This results in decreased physical fitness, which may eventually make fibromyalgia symptoms worse.

In fact, some health experts believe that poor diet and exercising habits may be linked to the onset of fibromyalgia, not just its continuation. Lack of exercise can weaken the immune system and the body as a whole. For instance, earlier in this chapter I mentioned research which hypothesized that "microtrauma" (a very slight injury or lesion) in deconditioned muscles could be a cause of fibromyalgia pain.

Many experts are currently debating the role exercise should play in fibromyalgia treatment—not only what kinds of exercise fibromyalgia victims should or should not do, but whether they should exercise at all. I believe that although fibromyalgia pain may discourage or limit daily activity, individuals with the syndrome should make a goal to remain as active as possible. Exercise is a great way to beat fatigue and depression often associated with fibromyalgia. I will discuss my exercise program, designed specifically for fibromyalgia patients, in Chapter 9. Also, see the Resource Guide for more information.

The other way to fight fatigue and build immunity is through a proper diet. Mary Moeller, L.P.N. and fibromyalgia survivor, writes in *The Fibromyalgia Nutrition Guide* (which I co-authored) that lack of proper nutrition and improper eating habits may cause many of the symptoms associated with fibromyalgia. The food we eat should provide us with all of the energy and nutrients we need for our bodies to function properly. If our immune system is compromised by stress and we are consuming foods with little nutritional value, we are not giving our bodies what they need to be healthy. Bodies compromised by stress and poor diet are more vulnerable to diseases. Fibromyalgia sufferers need to adopt healthy eating habits, not only for nutrition, but also to avoid potentially harmful food additives and preservatives that can lead to nutrient deficiencies, food allergies, depression and fatigue, among other things. Diet will be discussed in Chapter 6.

Vitamin and Mineral Deficiencies

Less than 10 percent of Americans eat a balanced diet, and more than half of the average person's daily calories come from foods like soft drinks and nutrient-deficient snacks. Deficiencies of various nutrients can cause a number of fibromyalgia symptoms, including depression, fatigue, confusion, insomnia, forgetfulness and anxiety. In fact, certain key nutrients are essential for the body to produce energy properly.

The Role of Magnesium in Energy Production

Some current research now indicates that fibromyalgia sufferers are deficient in certain compounds that are required for the body to produce energy. In fact, it is estimated that 72 *percent of Americans* don't even get the recommended daily allowance (RDA) of magnesium. The presence of magnesium, substrate oxygen, and phosphates are essential for energy production. High concentrations are required for healthy cellular respiration and the production of energy. On the other hand, deficiencies in these substances can seriously impede the Krebs cycle (human energy cycle), causing a reduction in the body's ability to utilize oxygen for muscle energy. A deficiency of the above factors very clearly leads to the symptoms of fatigue, depression and muscle pain in the fibromyalgia victims.

New research suggests that magnesium, being one of the most crucial elements for ATP synthesis, is usually below normal range when measured in fibromyalgia patients. Magnesium is one of the five ingredients required for the synthesis of ATP, which is necessary for energy and movement. (It is also interesting to note that most migraine headache victims suffer from a magnesium deficiency.)

The B-Complex Vitamins

Thiamin (B1), riboflavin (B2), and pyridoxine (B6) are essential for electron transport in the respiratory system. All three vitamins require a magnesium-dependent phosphate transferring action to become biologically active. When there is a magnesium deficiency, there is a breakdown in the body's energy production process. B vitamins are discussed in more detail in Chapter 8.

What About Aluminum?

It is now known that magnesium is also needed to help the body block toxic effects of aluminum; therefore, aluminum toxicity may play a role in symptoms experienced by magnesium-deficient fibromyalgia patients (Weintraub, 1997). Aluminum inhibits glycolysis (the production of energy) and oxidative phosphorylation (the conversion of ADP to ATP). Additionally, due to its high affinity for phosphate groups, aluminum blocks the absorption and utilization of phosphates that are critical to the creation of energy. The possible effects of aluminum toxicity on fibromyalgia sufferers needs to be acknowledged and addressed. Aluminum is discussed in more detail in Chapter 7.

Magnesium and Malic Acid

Since aluminum has been identified as a toxic metal leading to major metabolic disturbances, researchers have carefully studied means of eliminating it from the body's vital organs. It has been discovered that proper amounts of magnesium, along with supplemental malic acid, can act as a most potent aluminum detoxifier and are especially effective at decreasing aluminum toxicity in the vital organs of the body, especially the brain. Malic acid is effective because it has been shown to significantly increase the fecal and urinary secretion of aluminum, reducing the concentration of the metal found in the internal organs, tissues and the brain (Weintraub, 1997).

A research study done in 1992 shows the combined effects of malic acid and magnesium on fibromyalgia patients. Fifteen patients between the ages of thirty-two and sixty volunteered to participate in an open clinical setting where oral magnesium and malic acid preparations were ingested for a period of four to eight weeks. The patients ingested 1,200–2,400 milligrams of malic acid with 30–600 milligrams of magnesium. The results of the study are encouraging as all patients reported significant pain relief within just forty-eight hours of treatment. Results of studies such as this one gives us continuous hope for the fibromyalgia patient through nutritional and supplemental treatment (Abraham, 1992).

Manganese–A Critical Supplement

Recent studies have investigated the link between chronic fatigue syndrome and fibromyalgia syndrome, specifically why fatigue is one of the most prominent features in both syndromes. Many experts believe it may have something to do with manganese-dependent neuroendocrine (brain-hormone) changes, especially along the hypothalamic-pituitary-thyroid axis. Specifically, the cycle begins with the production of thyrotropin-releasing hormones (TRH) by the hypothalamus. TRH stimulates the pituitary gland to produce thyroid-stimulating hormones (TSH), which in turn stimulates production of thyroxin by the thyroid gland. This is critical simply because thyroxin regulates metabolic rate. Since fatigue is one of the primary conditions of both fibromyalgia and chronic fatigue victims, hypometabolism (decreased metabolism) due to secondary hypothyroidism may be to blame. And because manganese directly influences metabolic rate through its involvement in this hypothalamic-pituitary-thyroid axis, it may be a helpful mineral supplement for both fibromyalgia and chronic fatigue victims.

Those diagnosed with fibromyalgia should consider nutritional supplementation of magnesium, malic acid and manganese for the production of energy, for aluminum detoxification and to enhance metabolism in the recovery and return to general health and well-being. I discuss nutritional supplementation in further detail in Chapter 8.

2

Diagnosing Fibromyalgia

"We must cultivate our garden."
– VOLTAIRE

How Is Fibromyalgia Diagnosed?

Now that you have a better idea about the symptoms and possible causes of fibromyalgia, it is time to talk about how it is diagnosed. I've already mentioned the fact that when trying to diagnose fibromyalgia, normal laboratory testing will reveal very little or nothing. In other words, blood tests or x-rays are of no value, except in ruling out other illnesses—or what rheumatologist Roland Staud calls "a diagnosis of exclusion" (Remington, 2001). Fibromyalgia is only considered primary when its symptoms are not associated with other conditions such as trauma, cancer, thyroid disease or rheumatic arthritis. This fact initially led physicians to consider the problem described by these patients to be "in their heads," a form of masked depression or hypochondria. However, later research involving extensive physiological tests has shown that these impressions are untrue or unfounded. Below is a short list of other illnesses that must be ruled out when diagnosing fibromyalgia (or that can coexist with the disease). By looking at this list, it is easy to see how under- and overdiagnosis, as well as misdiagnosis, remain problems:

- candida overgrowth (yeast infection)
- carpal tunnel syndrome
- chronic fatigue syndrome (CFS)
- chronic infections
- depression or related psychological problems
- digestive and/or eating disorders, malabsorption
- drug side effects/chemical or food sensitivities
- hepatitis
- HIV/AIDS
- hormone imbalance or dysfunction
- hypoglycemia/diabetes
- hypothyroidism
- immune system dysfunction/autoimmune diseases
- irritable bowel syndrome (IBS)
- lupus
- lyme disease
- myofascial pain syndrome (MPS)
- osteoarthritis/rheumatoid arthritis
- seasonal affective disorder (SAD)
- sleep apnea or other sleep disorder
- temporomandibular joint disorder (TMJD)

After ruling out other illnesses, a diagnosis of fibromyalgia by health professionals or physicians is based on taking a careful personal or family history and by pinpointing tender areas in specific locations of muscle throughout the body called *tender points*. The criteria for fibromyalgia classification determined by the American College of Rheumatology in 1990 state that for the patient to be diagnosed as having the condition they must first, have "a history of widespread pain." The pain must be long-term and ongoing, and it is considered wide-

Fibromyalgia or Chronic Fatigue Syndrome?

A decade ago, many scientists believed that the only difference between the fibromyalgia and chronic fatigue syndrome patient was the degree of pain (Goldenberg, 1990) because about 75 percent of patients diagnosed with chronic fatigue syndrome meet the criteria of fibromyalgia syndrome (Buchwald, 1987), and until recently, many experts deemed it unlikely that these two conditions stemmed from separate disease processes. However, one recent study uncovered significant differences in homeostatic heart rate and blood pressure responses between fibromyalgia and chronic fatigue sufferers, which suggests that biological responses to stress in FM and CFS patients differ. Researchers in the study concluded that their findings "challenged the hypothesis that FM [fibromyalgia] and CFS [chronic fatigue syndrome] share a common derangement of the stress-response system" (Naschitz, 2001).

Another study (Buskila, 2001) found that cytokine (immune cell) abnormalities in fibromyalgia patients are not dominant in chronic fatigue patients, which suggests further differences between the two syndromes. And in a 2000 issue of *Current Review of Pain,* researchers noted that out of all subjects tested, only fibromyalgia sufferers experienced abnormal responses to mild stimulation. They list neuropeptide and brain activity differences that distinguish fibromyalgia from chronic fatigue (Bradley). These findings raise questions about the earlier belief that the only thing which differentiates the two is the degree of pain (Wolfe, 1993).

spread when it is present on the left *and* right sides of the body as well as above and below the waist. In addition, pain in the cervical spine, anterior chest, thoracic spine or lower back must also be present. Secondly, they must have pain in at least eleven of the eighteen tender points. Tender points must be painful to the touch, not just tender to the touch. One of the general

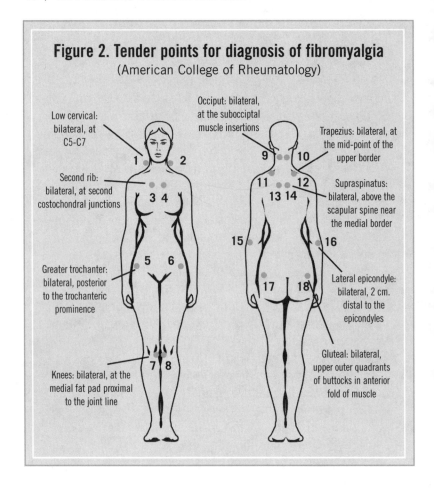

Figure 2. Tender points for diagnosis of fibromyalgia
(American College of Rheumatology)

Low cervical: bilateral, at C5-C7

Occiput: bilateral, at the subocciptal muscle insertions

Trapezius: bilateral, at the mid-point of the upper border

Second rib: bilateral, at second costochondral junctions

Supraspinatus: bilateral, above the scapular spine near the medial border

Greater trochanter: bilateral, posterior to the trochanteric prominence

Lateral epicondyle: bilateral, 2 cm. distal to the epicondyles

Gluteal: bilateral, upper outer quadrants of buttocks in anterior fold of muscle

Knees: bilateral, at the medial fat pad proximal to the joint line

guidelines followed for diagnostic criteria is a demonstration of widespread pain in all four quadrants of the body *for a minimum of three months*. (See Figure 2.)

A landmark study published in the February 1990 issue of *Arthritis and Rheumatism* provides further evidence to show the validity of fibromyalgia syndrome and diagnosis. The multicenter criteria study analyzed an experimental group of 558 patients; 265 were classified with fibromyalgia syndrome. The control group was not made up of typically healthy individuals. All the age and sex matched patients exhibited neck pain, low back pain, trauma-related pain syndromes, tendinitis, rheumatoid arthritis, lupus and other painful disorders. Each patient had some symptoms similar to those of fibromyalgia syndrome. Trained examiners were then asked to handpick those with fibromyalgia out of all subjects in the study. Results showed that these examiners were able to pinpoint fibromyalgia sufferers with *an accuracy rate of 88 percent* (Wolfe, 1990).

This study also illustrates why lab tests are important for those individuals who suspect they have fibromyalgia—to rule out several conditions that could be confused with fibromyalgia and to help avoid a misdiagnosis. For instance, an SED rate should be done on older patients to rule out *polymyalgia rheumatica*.

The Health Risk Appraisal Patient Profile

In order to determine whether a person has fibromyalgia, it is absolutely essential that time is taken to document a detailed history. With time constraints for today's physicians and health professionals, it becomes more and more essential to discover ways to be more efficient and to work smarter, and a thorough history is vital to proper diagnosis and patient care. This profile can be extremely helpful to the physician or healthcare practitioner attempting to diagnose and treat the potential fibromyalgia patient. It should include most of the following categories:

• Eating patterns (diet)
• Medications
• Sleep patterns and quality
• Fatigue frequency and intensity
• Pain and stiffness
• Swelling in soft tissue
• Accidents and illnesses
• Emotional trauma
• Allergies
• Family history

- Life history
- Functional history
- Perpetuating factors

The advantage of a detailed history form is that the patient can fill it out while in the waiting room at their doctor's office or use the one provided in this book to get a head start. (See Appendix A.) The doctor or health professional can then fill in the blanks during the initial interview. The patient will receive more thorough and efficient care and will save time.

Lab Tests to Consider if You Suspect Fibromyalgia

You may want to get the following done if you suspect fibromyalgia—if for no other reason than to rule out other illnesses and/or coexisting conditions. Don't be afraid to ask your doctor to explain the results and get copies for yourself of all results:

- Adrenal tests (including DHEA and cortisol)
- Autoimmune tests (for rheumatoid arthritis, gout, etc.)
- Blood sugar tests
- Candida yeast test
- CBC (complete blood count)
- Heavy metal or toxin exposure tests (hair analysis)
- HIV and hepatitis testing
- Hormone testing (estrogen, progesterone, testosterone, etc.)
- Parasite/malabsorption testing (stool analysis)
- Test for Lyme disease
- Tests for food and other allergies
- Thyroid testing

After Diagnosis: What Now?

Once you (and your doctor) have established fibromyalgia syndrome as the probable cause of your symptoms, it is a good idea to take stock of your resources. Is your current doctor going to work with you on treatment? Do you need to see a specialist? What kinds of additional research do you need to do as you construct a treatment plan? Are there support groups in your area or online that you can turn to for support? What role do you want friends and family to play? Are you going to use conventional or alternative therapies, or a combination of both?

In addition to answering these questions, it is a good idea to prioritize your health problems. Decide what you need to fix immediately and what can wait. It is also a good idea to start with the simplest and least aggressive/invasive treatments first. If you can treat a symptom with a simple change in diet—like giving up caffeine—why pay for a prescription drug that may have side effects? In fact, it is often a good idea to avoid prescription drugs as your primary form of treatment. These drugs often have side effects that can aggravate other symptoms.

In most cases, the best primary form of treatment that you can implement *immediately* after diagnosis is a change in lifestyle. Like other chronic conditions (diabetes, arthritis, irritable bowel syndrome), fibromyalgia symptoms can often be controlled, if not reversed, through simple diet and lifestyle changes that will be discussed throughout the book. And when you combine your change in lifestyle with other conventional and alternative therapies catered to your needs, fibromyalgia will lose its grip on your life. Even if you do experience flare-ups common among sufferers, they will not be as frequent or severe as they have been in the past. In fact, my using the techniques I outline in this book, you have the chance to reverse fibromyalgia completely and eradicate it from your life.

All that is required from you is an open mind, a willingness to change your current situation, and patience. You will see improvements in your symptoms and overall quality of life, but change will be gradual. Your fibromyalgia developed over time, and it will take time for it to fade. Because instant changes in your situation are not guaranteed, it is essential that you stick with it, believe in your ability to heal and preserve your hope for a pain-free future.

Examination and Treatment Plan for Fibromyalgia Patients

STEP 1: Patient Profile/Health Risk Appraisal

- Fill out the patient profile form (in Appendix A) before your first doctor visit.
- Have a doctor or health professional complete your profile during your interview.

STEP 2: Neurological, Joint and Musculoskeletal Evaluations

- Begin with the neurological evaluation.
- Then, start the joint evaluation to check for deformities, erythema and range of motion limitations.
- Finally, complete the musculoskeletal evaluation to test trigger points, gait, soft tissues and structural asymmetries.

STEP 3: Discuss Your Diagnosis and its Effects with Your Doctor

- Don't be afraid to involve your spouse and family in this segment of diagnosis.
- Educate yourself on what your diagnosis means.

STEP 4: Discuss Treatment Plans with your Doctor

- Understand how carbs, protein and fats should be balanced in your meals.
- Learn how to use menus and meal planning.
- Keep a food journal.
- Discuss the value of certain supplements in treatment.

• *Note:* See menus, food lists, meal planning forms, food journal examples, etc. in Chapter 6 and Appendix B.

STEP 5: The Importance of Sleep

• Learn techniques for returning to deep sleep.
• Begin keeping records of your sleeping habits.

STEP 6: Using Medication

• If possible, avoid steroids.
• If pain medication is necessary, use it only for short periods.
• If antidepressants are needed, discuss natural alternatives with your doctor.
• Review medications and supplements consistently.

STEP 7: Review Treatment Plans Periodically

• Continually educate yourself with books, handouts, videos, etc.
• Consider routine doctor visits every two to three weeks in the beginning.
• During acute rehab, see a specialist every four to eight weeks.
• Once your plan is established, review it every six months.
• Revamp your plan as needed for flare-ups.

Finding A Doctor

Finding the right doctor is imperative to successful fibromyalgia treatment. If you decide that your current primary care physician is not going to work for you—because they do not know enough about fibromyalgia or they are not open to alternative treatments—one of the first things you must do once you are diagnosed is find a doctor who will be your partner in developing a treatment plan. The ideal candidate would be a doctor who recognizes the validity of fibromyalgia and is familiar with it. He (or she) should also be open to a variety of treatments and consider you an equal partner in deciding treatment. If you feel rushed or ignored, move on! You need a physician who will listen and who you will feel comfortable with.

If you are starting from scratch, it is often a good idea to find doctors based on referrals and word of mouth. Sometimes fibromyalgia support organizations will list doctors familiar with fibromyalgia, or you can contact the American College of Rheumatology. I also have collected some fibromyalgia resources located in the back of the book that may help.

Once you find a doctor, ask them for endorsements, check their schooling and question them about their level of experience with fibromyalgia. It is also a good idea to ask them whether they are comfortable and willing to work with other healthcare professionals—like an acupuncturist or nutritionist—because you will probably need the help of more than one person if you want your treatment to be successful. Your doctor's willingness to work as a team will also help you get referrals to other helpful healthcare workers that will help you with your health insurance provider.

On your first visit, you should also prepare by writing down the reasons for your visit, questions for your doctor, and what you expect from him during the visit and over the long haul. It is also a good idea to keep a daily symptom journal where you right down any information you feel will help your doctor with treatment. Be as specific as possible. Don't just write down your symptoms, but also the time you felt symptoms, your level of daily activity, what you ate and did, and anything in your routine that may account for flare-ups—stress, changes in routine, weather changes, etc. Anything that may be a trigger should be written down. If you are taking herbal supplements, vitamins or prescription, or over-the-counter drugs for fibromyalgia (or any other reason), you should also make a list of these items for your doctor. You may be experiencing side effects or adverse drug interactions (or drug-herb interactions).

"I noticed an amazing difference"

I was diagnosed with vasculitis and peripheral neuropathy in 1994. I was in severe pain and was on steroids for five years, along with other drugs. But the pain continued, and I began developing fibromyalgia symptoms along with the other pain and problems. I had taken countless natural products and had never had any positive results from anything.

Then I read Dr. Elrod's book about reversing fibromyalgia. I faxed him a note about where to get these supplements he was describing in the book. He began to tell me about the great products that had been developed for people like me with aches, pain, sleeping disorders, etc. After following his advice, I noticed an amazing difference after three weeks. I could not believe it.

That was almost two years ago, and I have felt wonderful. The pain is gone and I have an abundance of energy. I am so grateful that Dr. Elrod took the time to call me back! What a change it has made in my life.

Stephanie B.
Spearman, Texas

Going Beyond Your Physician

Below is a list of other specialists that may also treat fibromyalgia patients. Often successful treatment depends on collaboration with various health care professionals. Each specialist will give you a unique perspective on your disease and how to treat it:

- chiropractor
- herbalist/naturopathic doctor
- massage therapist/acupuncturist (or acupressurist)
- medical researchers
- nurses

- nutritionist/dietician
- pharmacist/health food store educational specialist
- physical therapist
- psychiatrist, psychologist or other therapist
- rheumatologist

A Fallacy: Fibromyalgia Cannot Be Cured

The chronic problems of musculoskeletal pain and fatigue are common afflictions that most doctors believe are incurable. Generally, the patient is simply told that the pain is somewhat manageable through the use of drugs and therapy, but they are destined to live with this condition for the rest of their life. This is absolutely *not* true. The fibromyalgia reversal model found in this book has been developed over the past ten years and has helped many victims reverse the condition and return to vibrant, productive, healthy lives. The success stories found throughout the book reveal what the program has done for others and what it may do for you.

3

Traditional Treatments
for Fibromyalgia

*"Drugs are not always necessary, [but] belief in
recovery always is."* – NORMAN COUSINS

Once diagnosed with fibromyalgia, most patients receiving
medical advice from their family doctor will probably find
that the options they are given for treatment are limited and
often become ineffective over time. Traditional treatments for
fibromyalgia should not be disregarded and may be helpful, but
on their own, they usually do not offer sufferers the complete
and permanent relief they are looking for. The reason traditional treatments rarely work by themselves is because they are
geared primarily toward partial relief of symptoms, and since
they do not treat possible causes, they cannot cure fibromyalgia.

Conventional fibromyalgia treatments have evolved over the
years but have traditionally been geared toward using drugs to
reduce pain and increase the quality of sleep. Many doctors
focus on treating the sleep disorders common in fibromyalgia
patients because they are thought to be a major contributing
factor to the symptoms of the condition. The primary medications that have been prescribed for fibromyalgia are painkillers

and drugs that boost the body's level of a neurotransmitter known as serotonin which affects sleep, pain sensation and immune system function. Overall, this treatment method has not been very effective and, as a result, the treatment of fibromyalgia has been frustrating for both patients and physicians (Norregaard, 1995).

The major problem with drug treatments is that often, instead of getting to the source of the problem, they merely mask the symptoms. Also, there are almost always side effects, and very often these side effects can exacerbate the original problem and/or cause other problems that are as serious as the original condition. Furthermore, drug therapies aren't effective for everyone. Although general effects and side effects of a particular drug are known based on the results of scientific studies, drugs affect each person differently and often provide only partial and temporary relief. For example, a 2000 study in the *Journal of General Internal Medicine* found antidepressants to be effective for treating pain, fatigue and insomnia associated with fibromyalgia, but only in 25 percent of fibromyalgia patients tested, and researchers were not sure how long beneficial results would last. Furthermore, no effect on fibromyalgia trigger points was noted (O'Malley).

To boost the effectiveness of drug treatments, current accepted medical treatments for fibromyalgia often combine nondrug therapies with pain medication and antidepressants. For instance, medical practitioners give advice on stress management and often encourage patients to begin an exercise program (Littlejohn, 2001). Usually aerobic exercise programs are used since there has been increasing evidence that a regular program is essential for fibromyalgia patients. In the past, physicians and health professionals have taken fibromyalgia victims off exercise programs because the repetitive movements and exertion can sometimes increase pain and fatigue, making exercise quite difficult (McCain, 1988). However, as mentioned previously, inactivity may also cause fibromyalgia symptoms to worsen, and so an exercise program of some sort is often advised to treat and prevent depression, pain and fatigue associated with the syndrome. Chapter 9 discusses exercise options in more detail.

Other nondrug treatments that have been used over the years include trigger point injections with lidocaine (a local anesthetic), physical therapy, psychotherapy, acupressure, acupuncture, and techniques such as muscle relaxation, breathing exercises, osteopathic manipulation and therapeutic massage, some of which I will discuss in more detail later in the book.

Although nondrug and alternative therapies are very useful, there are times when pain relievers may be necessary, and your physician will probably prescribe some (Jaeschke, 1991). Don't be afraid to take prescribed medication when necessary, but it is important that you don't rely on it daily. Choose natural treatment over drug treatment when possible. It is also important that before taking any medication, you understand what it is supposed to do and what the side effects may be. Explore the various types of medications that are used to treat fibromyalgia, and don't be afraid to talk to your doctor about changing medications that aren't effective or cause problems. I very strongly recommend that you follow your physician's advice when taking the medications prescribed for your condition, but it is my sincere hope that you will be able to move toward a more natural regimen. By combining the most effective therapies from mainstream and natural medicine, it is my belief that you can overcome fibromyalgia and lead a healthy, pain-free life.

Drugs Used to Treat Fibromyalgia

To construct the best possible fibromyalgia treatment plan, it is important to understand what traditional medications can do and what the risks are. Once you know both your conventional and alternative treatment options, you will be better prepared to make important decisions about your health. Let's look at the various drug categories and specific drugs that have been used in traditional treatment of fibromyalgia, some of the problems associated with the drugs, and what to expect based on the accumulated research (Bennet, Goldenberg, and McCain).

"It is a very practical and powerful program!"

After having read your book, for the first time in years I have some hope for my life. I was first diagnosed with this painful condition about fifteen years ago—three years after an accident which left me in severe pain and no medical explanation other than it must be "in my head." Since I was in a 12-step recovery program for drug addiction, I chose to no longer take the pain killers, muscle relaxants and good old amitriptyline (which induced a very different side effect in me—I became VERY suicidal). The spinal manipulations, massage and acupuncture treatments work fairly well for me, but since my insurance no longer covers these treatments, I can't afford to pay for them. I have started several exercise programs, only to begin the pain and muscle spasm cycle again. I feel so very helpless, which has led to severe depression which starts yet another cycle of pain and muscle spasms. It seems to be the same cycle of everyone I've ever known with fibromyalgia.

Your book has offered me hope to have more of a real life now. I fully believe in the mind and body to have to work together to overcome any kind of disease and you have put it all into one volume! It is a very practical and powerful program!

Thank you so very much for having such compassion for those of us who are inflicted with this challenge and going the extra mile to put a program together for us which we can follow and lead a much more productive life. God Bless You,

Fern L.
Arkansas

Antidepressants

As mentioned earlier, antidepressants are often prescribed to treat symptoms of insomnia, fatigue, pain and depression in fibromyalgics. Typically, antidepressants fall into one of three categories: tricyclics or tetracyclics, monoamine oxidase inhibitors (MAOIs) and selective serotonin re-uptake inhibitors (SSRIs). Each of the three types alters brain chemistry in a particular way without being addictive. Tricyclics increase the brain's exposure to serotonin, and the tricyclic Elavil (amitriptyline) is sometimes prescribed for fibromyalgia. MAOIs influence the neurotransmitters known as monoamines—serotonin, norepinephrine and dopamine. MAOIs commonly prescribed for fibromyalgics include Nardil (phenelzine) and Parnate (tranylcypromine). SSRIs like Prozac (fluoxetine), Paxil (paroxetine) and Zoloft (sertraline) are also commonly used in the treatment of fibromyalgia and increase the brain's exposure to serotonin as well. Flexeril (cyclobenzaprine), Xanax (alprazolam) and klonopin are also sometimes prescribed.

Despite the links between fibromyalgia symptoms and serotonin levels, research shows that less than half of fibromyalgics tested actually experience significant, long-term relief by using only antidepressants. The amount of improvement can vary greatly from person to person. Furthermore, antidepressant have no effect on trigger point pain, and side effects associated with antidepressant are numerous. The side effects of tricyclics include rapid heartbeat, high blood pressure, heart attack stroke, hallucinations, confusion, anxiety, nightmares, insomnia, numbness, tingling and headaches. The MAO inhibitor Nardil is associated with impaired B6 production. (Vitamin B6 deficiencies are associated with depression and PMS.) And SSRIs can cause decreased libido, memory loss, insomnia, erratic behavior, mood swings and headaches as. Other side effects of antidepressants include dry mouth, daytime drowsiness, increased appetite and constipation. Although these side effects are rarely severe, they can be disturbing and may limit the use of the drugs (Russell, 1991). Some side effects, like insomnia, may even complicate or worsen fibromyalgia symptoms.

Sleeping Pills

It is also very important to avoid prescription tranquilizers and sleeping medications of the benzodiazepine group. While these may help or assist sleep, they suppress deep sleep and often make fibromyalgia symptoms worse. If your doctor wants to prescribe sleeping pills for you, for your own sake, decline. The routine use of sleeping pills such as valium, halcion and restoril not only impair the quality of deep sleep, they can also be addictive.

Corticosteroids

Powerful drugs such as prednisone and cortisone are corticosteroids (adrenal-cortex steroids) that are sometimes prescribed for severe pain. These anti-inflammatory agents are excellent at reducing fibromyalgia pain but have some very serious side effects that put them in the "dangerous" category. Some of the side effects are thinning of the bones and increased risk of bone fractures, impairment of wound healing and depression of the immune system. When taken in large doses over long periods of time, corticosteroids can also cause osteoporosis, diabetes and hypertension. They have been reported to cause mental disturbances.

Corticosteroids can also interfere with proper nutrition. They may potentially decrease the absorption of vitamin D, causing water retention and enhancing the rate of excretion of vitamin C, potassium and zinc. Should you choose to take prescribed corticosteroids, it would be wise to increase dosage of these nutrients. The good news is that, once you get into your fibromyalgia cure regimen, the need for these nutritionally disturbing medications will be lessened or eliminated (Brooks and Day, 1991).

Acetaminophen and NSAIDs

Because of the risks associated with corticosteroids, NSAIDs were developed as alternatives (Calabro, 1992). Acetaminophen and NSAIDs (nonsteroidal anti-inflammatory drugs) are prescribed to treat similar symptoms. Acetaminophen is sold under the trade names Tylenol, Liquiprin and Datril. Some of the common nonsteroidal anti-inflammatory drugs are sold under the names of Motrin, Advil and aspirin.

It is important to point out the differences between acetaminophen and NSAIDs. Both are prescribed as pain relievers and do an excellent job. However, acetaminophen is an analgesic and an antipyretic, which means that it relieves pain and lowers fever. Nonsteroidal anti-inflammatory drugs help reduce fever, fight pain and remove inflammation. Some physicians will opt for prescribing acetaminophen since it is less expensive and has fewer side effects than the NSAIDs. However, do not be misled because acetaminophen certainly has its own side effects (Gay, 1990). According to Sandler (1989), acetaminophen is well tolerated and safe if taken in a standard dosage of below four grams per twenty-four hour period. However, if taken over a long period of time, acetaminophen carries the danger of a small but significant decrease in liver function and possesses a possibility for harming the kidneys. In the Harvard *Health Letter*, Garnett (1995) suggests taking precautions with acetaminophen as studies and research show that it is probably the culprit in as many as 5,000 cases of kidney failure in the United States annually.

What about NSAIDs?

Aspirin is by far the most popular and best known of the NSAIDs. It belongs to a class of drugs called salicylates used to treat osteoarthritis, various forms of rheumatism and many other kinds of pain for more than a hundred years. Small doses are typically used to treat pain while larger doses are generally prescribed for inflammation. In the 1960s, other NSAIDs such as indomethacin (indocin) were developed, followed by ibuprofen. The development of NSAIDs has continued, and currently there are more than one hundred different nonsteroidal anti-inflammatory drugs either on the market or under investigation for approval. Nonprescription, over-the-counter NSAIDs include the brand names Excedrin, Midol, Nuprin, Advil, Aleve and Motrin.

Nonsteroidal anti-inflammatory drugs work primarily by impeding the production of prostaglandins, hormone substances in the body that enhance pain and inflammation responses. Prostaglandins, however, are also necessary in various body functions, such as the regulation of blood pressure, blood coagulation, the secretion of gastric juices in the stomach and kidney regulation. As one would suspect, drugs that interfere with the negative actions of prostaglandins will also affect their positive purposes as well. So although they are often a better choice that corticosteroids, NSAIDs have a large number of side effects that interfere with bodily functions due to its negative effects on prostaglandins (Novak, 1995). Some of the common and potentially serious side effects are:

- nausea
- indigestion
- constipation
- nervousness
- drowsiness
- ulcers/stomach bleeding
- weight gain
- urinary problems
- intestinal cramps
- diarrhea
- sensitivity to sunlight
- confusion
- headache
- high blood pressure
- swelling of hands/feet
- sore throat/fever

Another side effect that is more rare is *anaphylaxis*, a severe allergic reaction characterized by difficulty in breathing or swallowing, a swollen tongue, dizziness, fainting, hives, puffy eyelids, fast and irregular heartbeat, and a change in face color. You should immediately seek help if you experience any of these signs after taking NSAIDs.

So while NSAIDs can be quite helpful when used on a short-term basis to relieve pain, they can be very harmful when used over long periods because though the pain is relieved, the underlying disease condition continues. NSAIDs do not cure disease, so disease processes continue whether the patient feels the effects or not (Hendler 1992). In a five-year clinical study, Hodgkinson and Woolf (1979) reported that NSAIDs did not delay the progression of chronic pain diseases. In fact, they actually hastened their progress in some cases. And Dr. Paul St. Amand, author of *What Your Doctor May Not Tell You about Fibromyalgia* (1999), believes that salicylates like aspirin are the worst thing that fibromyalgics can take. Instead, he suggests a regimen with guaifenesin, a drug often used to treat colds and allergies.

Furthermore, as Dr. Theodosakis (1997) points out, while NSAIDs generally provide faster pain relief than natural supplements, the pain relief quickly plateaus and often diminishes with time. If pain and symptoms are severe, you may want to use pain relievers in conjunction with natural treatments and then taper off the medication as the nutritional supplements begin to aid your total condition. Naturally, these adjustments would have to occur with the approval and under the direction of your physician or healthcare provider.

How Should I Treat NSAID Side Effects?

Stehlin (1990) suggests the following guidelines for lessening the side effects of NSAIDs:

- In general, all NSAIDs should be taken with food. It's often helpful to eat, take the pill, and then eat again.
- In order to control the development of ulcers while you're taking NSAIDs, your doctor may prescribe Misoprostol. If you are pregnant, your doctor will suggest a different medication.
- Drink at least eight ounces of water when taking tablets or capsules to keep the lining of the esophagus and stomach from becoming irritated.
- Don't lie down for thirty minutes or so after taking your medicine. Gravity helps assure that the pill passes through the esophagus.
- Always take the exact dose prescribed by your doctor. Never double it, even if you miss a scheduled dose.
- Pregnant or breast-feeding women should not take NSAIDs unless specifically directed to by a doctor.
- Do not use alcohol while taking NSAIDs. Doing so increases the risk of stomach problems.
- Don't combine acetaminophen (such as Tylenol) with NSAIDs unless specifically directed to do so by your doctor.
- Inform your doctor of all other medications you are taking, whether prescription or over-the-counter, so it can be determined whether one drug will interact with another. Also, it never hurts to double-check drug interactions on your own, especially if you are taking herbs and supplements, which your doctor may have limited or outdated knowledge about.
- If you are having surgery, inform your doctor or dentist that you are on NSAID therapy, even a low dose.
- Avoid driving or operating machinery when you are taking NSAIDs because they may cause drowsiness, confusion or dizziness in a small number of patients.
- Avoid direct sunlight. Your skin is more sensitive to sunlight during NSAID therapy.

Suggestions for Taking Medications

Physicians make the very best decisions that they possibly can, but in many cases it is very difficult to prescribe the proper medication with the right dose to be taken at the right time for the right reasons. Physicians may be unaware of some of the side effects of medications, or they may not be aware of the drug history of a patient, or they aren't told what drugs may have been prescribed alongside other drugs being suggested at any particular time. Also, many physicians are now required to prescribe from a limited number of drugs, even if another one may be better suited for your needs.

These are all very good reasons for you to be well informed and educated about the medications that may be prescribed for you. Also be sure that your physician has a complete history of any drugs that you have used or are currently taking. The following are some guidelines and questions to ask as you work with your physician on the proper regimen for prescriptions:

• Why do I need this drug?
• What are the possible side effects—from the most common to the most rare?
• Who is most likely to suffer from the side effects of this drug?
• What are the early warning signs of side effects associated with this drug?
• Are there any serious health risks associated with taking this drug?
• Is there another medicine better suited to my needs?
• Is there a generic version of the drug that would work just as well for me but cost less?
• How many times a day should I take the medication? When? Should I take it with food or water, or on an empty stomach?
• Are there any foods or drinks I should avoid while taking this drug?
• Are there any medications, supplements or herbs I should avoid while on this medication?

- Are there any activities I should restrict or avoid doing while using this drug?
- How long will I have to take the drug before I can tell whether or not it is working?
- How will I know it's working?
- Assuming it works, how long should I continue taking it? If I do not like the drug's effects (or lack of) can I discontinue use on my own or do I need to consult a doctor before discontinuing?
- What should I do if I accidentally skip a scheduled dose?
- Is this a drug I must take daily or can I take it as needed?
- If it doesn't work, how long before we try something else?
- Is there a nondrug treatment I might try instead or that can be used in conjunction with this drug?

Be certain that your physician is aware of your complete regimen, including your diet, the nutritional supplements you're taking, and any other drugs or herbal remedies that you are currently taking. If your physician prescribes medications for your condition, ask about supplemental nutrients. If your doctor does not know all the answers to your questions, don't be afraid to ask your pharmacist or another healthcare provider. Some research you can even do on your own on your computer or at the library.

Nondrug Therapies

As mentioned at the start of this chapter, mainstream medicine also uses a number of nondrug treatments for fibromyalgia sufferers. Except for dietary or supplement therapies, such treatments usually fall into one of two categories: physical therapies (PT) or mind-body therapies (MBT). Exercise (PT) and counseling (MBT) are both great examples of nondrug treatments often suggested by doctors for treating fibromyalgia. Below is a short list of other nondrug treatments–some more conventional than others—that may be helpful. This is by no means a complete list of treatments available, but it should give you an idea of some of the options out there:

Acupressure/Acupuncture

Using acupuncture and acupressure to treat fibromyalgia is still under debate. Some fibromyalgics swear by it, but others say that it just makes the pain worse. According to a 1999 review of various complementary medical treatments, acupuncture is one of three complementary and alternative medicine (CAM) therapies that is supported by empirical research. Reviewers found "moderately strong" support for acupuncture treatment of fibromyalgia, but said that for some patients, acupuncture will only "exacerbate symptoms" and further complicate the condition (Berman).

A more recent review concluded that "acupuncture may reduce pain and increase pain threshold" in fibromyalgia patients, and an approach that combines various physical therapies like acupuncture is a "promising strategy" for treating fibromyalgia (Offenbacher, 2000).

These therapies may be used to counteract symptoms of chronic pain, depression, anxiety, insomnia, headaches, stress, digestive distress and menstrual problems associated with fibromyalgia. Some people even use acupuncture to help them quit smoking. Along with traditional acupressure and acupuncture, there a number of variations on these therapies. For instance, some practitioners may apply warm bundles of herbs to acupuncture points instead of or along with needles. And some practitioners use electrical currents instead of needles. In fact, some fibromyalgics may achieve better results with electroacupuncture, according to research. For those who choose acupressure, there are many techniques that may be done on your own, without the help of an acupressurist, if you learn how to do them properly.

Perhaps the greatest determining factor in the success of failure of these treatments is the experience of the practitioner. Inexperienced acupuncturists (or acupressurists) or those not familiar with fibromyalgia may do more harm than good. Make sure you find someone who is properly trained and licensed. Don't be afraid to ask for references before deciding to undergo treatment. For help if locating an experienced practitioner, contact the American Association of Oriental Medicine or related organizations.

Balneotherapy

Balneotherapy means "therapeutic baths," and it is a subset of hydrotherapy treatments. A 2001 study in *Clinical Rheumatology* studied the effects of balneotherapy on fibromyalgics' quality of life. Nearly fifty sufferers participated, and half received therapy at a spa that offered balneotherapy at the Dead Sea, while the other half did not. Before beginning, researchers assessed all participants for psychological well-being and fibromyalgia symptoms. Individuals who participated in the therapy stayed for ten days at the spa. They were assessed at the end of their stay, one month later and then a three-month follow-up. Those individuals who received the spa treatment reported less symptoms and better quality of life than those who did not receive treatment. The physical benefits of balneotherapy lasted for up to three months in most spa participants, but psychological improvements were more short-term. Researchers concluded that balneotherapy at the Dead Sea spa may provide transient improvement in fibromyalgics (Neumann).

Biofeedback

In Chapter 1, I discussed the stress link to fibromyalgia. Some researchers believe that the autonomic nervous system, which governs involuntary processes like blood pressure and temperature, is negatively affected when the body is exposed to long-term stress. If these processes are altered in the fibromyalgia sufferer because of chronic stress or a series of traumatic events, some scientists ask, is their a way to train the nervous system to be healthy again?

Neal Miller, the originator of biofeedback, believed that there was a way and began research in the the 1960s to prove it. Biofeedback focuses on the power of the mind in perpetuating and reversing disease. With the help of a biofeedback therapist, patients learn to modify their mental processes in ways that positively affect the autonomic nervous system and ultimately, temper or reverse chronic illnesses.

How does biofeedback work? Specialists in this mind-body approach use monitoring equipment to give the patient feedback on involuntary processes they may be unaware of. For example, biofeedback can be used to monitor blood pressure, temperature, and brain wave activity, among other things. The information is obtained using electrodes attached to areas that are being monitored. The information is carried to monitors and interpreted by a biofeedback specialist. The patient then uses the information to educate themselves on mental exercises and techniques they can use to positively influence health. Biofeedback not only increases body-mind awareness in patients, it also empowers them and encourages them to take a more active role in their health.

Biofeedback comes in many forms. Some measure muscle tension (EMG feedback), while others measure brain waves (EEG feedback). Still others measure temperature, electrical conductance, stomach acid, and respiration. There are currently more than 10,000 practitioners in the United States, and biofeedback is used for a variety of complaints, including stress, depression, irritable bladder, irritable bowel syndrome, alcohol or drug addiction, sleeping disorders, migraine or tension headaches, muscle dysfunction, and anxiety.

Biofeedback is also being used to treat fibromyalgia. A 1999 study out of Germany found that EMG biofeedback reduced pain and muscle tension in fibromyalgics, and also improved sleep and lowered headache occurrences (Mur). Another study published in *Arthritis Care Research* found that biofeedback and relaxation training, when combined with exercise, reduced tender point pain in sufferers when compared to the control group (who received education about the syndrome but not therapies). Individuals in the biofeedback-exercise group also maintained the benefits longer than those who did either biofeedback or exercise, but not both (Buckelew, 1998).

Furthermore, a 2001 study in the *Journal of Clinical Psychology* found that EEG biofeedback could potentially improve mental clarity, mood and sleep in clinically diagnosed fibromyalgia sufferers. EEG feedback also helped patients better determine the exact locations of their pain, which enabled them to get more beneficial pain treatment (Mueller).

Collagen Hydrolysat

Collagen hydrolysat, a food supplement available without a prescription, is currently being tested for its effectiveness in treating the symptoms of fibromyalgia and temporomandibular joint pain. Results published in an April 2000 issue of *Cranio* state that the supplement decreased pain significantly in some individuals and dramatically reduced pain in others.

Twenty diagnosed fibromyalgics were evaluated. All participants had been diagnosed for at least two years. Individuals were evaluated at the beginning of the evaluation, and then after thirty, sixty and ninety days. Researchers noted that the average pain complaints in participants dropped in the overall group, and for some, the beneficial effects of collagen hydrolysat were even more dramatic. They concluded that the supplement—which had no reported side effects—may be helpful for fibromyalgics, especially those with TMJ problems (Olson). More supplements are discussed in Chapter 8.

Magnets

Although there is a lot of debate over the credibility of magnet therapy, some researchers are finding magnetic sleep pads useful for treating fibromyalgia symptoms. One 2001 study evaluated fibromyalgics over a six-month period—some using magnetic sleep pads and others using sleep pads without active magnets. Those using the active magnetic pads experienced improvements in pain intensity and tender point pain, but tender point pain improvement was also noted in the control group (those not using active magnets). Decreases in pain intensity levels, however, were only significant in the magnet-treated group. Fibromyalgics may experience pain reduction from long-term use of magnetic sleep pads, but researchers are not sure whether the pads actually affect trigger point pain (Alfano).

Meditation (and Visual Imaging)

A May 2001 report from Reuters Health stated that meditation may alleviate symptoms of pain, fatigue and poor sleep in fibromyalgics. This finding is based on a study presented at the annual meeting of the American Psychosomatic Society in California. Ninety women with fibromyalgia participated in the study. Some were assigned to a four-month meditation stress-reduction program, and the others remained on a waiting list and did not participate in the program. The program helped women develop a daily routine of meditating for approximately one hour six days a week. The meditation programs were developed at the University of Massachusetts Medical School.

In order to test participants stress levels, researchers obtained saliva samples from the women during the study. From these samples and interviews with the women, researchers found that women who meditated daily lowered their cortisol levels, and were less depressed and slept better than those who did not meditate. These women also said that they felt fibromyalgia had less of a hold on their lives.

Researchers concluded that meditation could potentially reduce stress in fibromyalgics and perhaps even change the way

Prolotherapy for Fibromyalgia

Although prolotherapy is practiced by several hundred doctors in the United States, including former U.S. Surgeon General C. Everett Koop, it is still considered a controversial treatment by many in the mainstream medical community. Prolotherapy involves injecting a solution of a local anesthetic, dextrose (corn sugar) and Sarapin (a plant extract that soothes nerves) into the joints or trigger points of treated individuals.

The therapy may be used by those with back pain, migraines, osteoarthritis, tennis elbow, TMJ, tendinitis and fibromyalgia. And depending on the severity of the problem, patients may just need one session or a hundred. In addition, the treatment is covered by many insurance companies (but not Medicare).

How does prolotherapy work? Proponents believe that prolotherapy promotes healing by encouraging inflammation, rather than discouraging it as standard treatments like ice packs and ibuprofen do. Furthermore, prolotherapists hypothesize that many conditions for which the treatment is used can be traced back to the same cause, loose ligaments. Injections stimulate growth factors, which aid in ligament and tendon repair. Prolotherapy may also promote cartilage growth in the joint.

Skeptics of the therapy believe that to link weak ligaments to all joint pain is premature and overly simplified. Although ligament weakness can be connected to arthritis, links to headaches and fibromyalgia are unfounded. Skeptics also argue against the pro-inflammation theory of prolotherapists, saying that injections probably cause scar tissue to form, which is not a long-term solution for joint pain and joint health.

The biggest argument against using prolotherapy is the lack of research. Only a handful of scientifically sound studies have been done to test its effectiveness. However, the majority of these studies have found benefits to prolotherapy. One of the most recent of these studies was published in 2000 and found that prolotherapy could benefit those with knee osteoarthritis, especially with pain, swelling, knee buckling and flexibility (Reeves).

Studies accurately testing the effectiveness of prolotherapy on fibromyalgia are still lacking, but anecdotal evidence supports its possible use of fibromyalgia symptoms. If you do choose to try prolotherapy, be careful about choosing a doctor to perform the injections. Although complications are rare, improper injections may result in infection, spinal injury or even paralysis or death.

the body reacts to stressful events. In fact, the effects of one hour of meditation not only exist while meditating, they affect individuals for the other twenty-three hours as well. Researchers do warn, however, that these effects only work for individuals dedicated to regular and rigorous meditation daily.

Meditation (and visual imaging) are discussed in more detail in the next chapter.

Therapeutic Massage

As with acupuncture, treating fibromyalgia with massage can be tricky. Some medical practitioners find it helps their patients, but others believe that it aggravates symptoms. I believe that certain types of massage may be beneficial, but there are some factors you should consider before seeking treatment.

The most important, and I cannot overemphasize this, is choosing a licensed massage therapist with experience treating fibromyalgia symptoms. Massage therapy has the potential to alleviate complaints like chronic and short-term muscle and joint pain and stiffness, headaches, digestive complaints and even sinus problems, but only if it is done properly. As with acupuncturists, get references before starting treatment. Also, let the massage therapist know what other treatments you are undergoing.

Although more research on the benefits of massage need to be done, a recent review of physical therapies like massage found that "massage may reduce muscle tension and may be prescribed as an adjunct with other therapeutic interventions" (Offenbacher, 2000). But an earlier review done in 1999 found the scientific support for manipulative therapies like chiropractic and massage was weak and inconclusive.

As with acupuncture, there are many variations on standard massage that may be useful to you. A short list of these include: craniosacral release, trigger point therapy, and myofascial release. Another technique is called electrostatic massage, which uses static electricity. Ask your massage therapist about these and other options.

I believe that nondrug treatments are very helpful in the treatment of fibromyalgia, especially when combined to fit individual needs. However, I must end with a word of caution. Many CAM treatments have not been thoroughly tested, and new ones are popping up all the time. If you decide to use one or more of these treatments, please talk to at least one reliable experienced health profession before beginning. If you are careful and observant, you increase the likelihood of safe and effective treatment. To read a more thorough review on CAM treatments, refer to the April 2001 article "Complementary and Alternative Therapies for Fibromyalgia" in *Current Rheumatology Reports*.

4

The Mind-Body Connection

"Each patient carries his own doctor inside him."
– ALBERT SCHWEITZER

"I have learned never to underestimate the capacity of the human mind and body to regenerate—even when prospects seem most wretched. The life force may be the least understood force on this earth." – DR. NORMAN COUSINS

In the previous chapter, I discussed the value of traditional treatments and how they can be combined with alternative treatments for better results. My plan for reversing fibromyalgia is introduced in the next chapter, but before I discuss the specifics of the plan, I think it is important to mention the relationship between the mind and body that is often overlooked in traditional medicine. It is true that fibromyalgia is *not* "all in your head"—the symptoms are real and the pain is very real. But it is also true that the mind plays a very real role in our health.

In the second century, the Greek physician Galan noted that disease is a consequence of psychic imbalance. For more than a millennium that belief prevailed in the practice of medicine, until modern medical science rejected the idea that mental and emotional states influence the body's disease-fighting capacity.

However, about twenty-five years ago, the connection between physiological factors and immune functions was revived and seriously examined. In fact, the belief that this connection exists has birthed the field of investigation called psychoneuroimmunology (PNI) that is growing in popularity. PNI scholars and researchers focus primarily on how the brain and the body's immune system communicate.

PNI research indicates that vital body systems, the brain and the immune system, communicate with and influence one another. For instance, if your brain allows stress levels to get out of control, this can have a seriously detrimental impact on the immune system, which in turn can suppress its ability to fight disease. In other words, if you are chronically distressed, anxious or uptight, these emotions can manifest themselves over time as heart disease, cancer, arthritis, and even fibromyalgia. On the other hand, well-managed stress can help keep your immune system healthy. If we are well adjusted, happy and content, our bodies will maintain their disease-fighting forces at peak capacity.

The hypothalamus (the brain's autonomic center) and the pituitary gland (the body's master gland) are connected by a rich network of blood vessels. The discovery of this network has helped researchers understand how thoughts and emotions affect the immune system. The fact that stress hormones directly influence the immune response has been suspected for years by immunologists. Several research studies in recent years have indicated positive links between immune response and emotional factors. Research has also borne out that people being described as helpless, sad, unassertive, hopeless, passive, and fearful have shown greater incidences of cancer.

Communication between the brain and the immune system is fundamental. The lymph nodes, one of the immune systems principal groups of organs, are filled with nerve fibers that act like telephone trunk lines and send and receive messages for the entire body. Special chemicals called "neurotransmitters" attach themselves to immune cells and influence their disease-fighting potential.

Psychoneuroimmunology researcher, Dr. Candace Pert, contends that small protein-like brain chemicals called neuropeptides provide the chemical basis of emotion. Neuropeptides have powerful mood stimulating effects, and high concentrations of them are found in the limbic system of the brain, thought to be the "control center" of emotions. Endorphins, which are two hundred times more powerful than morphine, are examples of neuropeptides.

Intense and persistent periods of negative emotions such as fear, depression, grieving and helplessness have been shown to suppress normal immune functions. On the other hand, research has shown that we can strengthen the immune system with confidence, happiness, laughter and other positive emotions. To achieve the highest level of health that we are capable of reaching, we absolutely need to establish a positive thought structure as our normal daily attitude. This program is designed to assist you in achieving just that.

Why would mother nature link negative stress with the immune system? There are several possible explanations that have been offered by immunologists. One widely accepted theory points to energy preservation. Temporarily diverting energy away from the constant struggles of the immune system commits more energy to the perceived threat outside signaled by stress hormones. The greater the perceived "threat" and the negative emotion, the greater the degree of immune suppression. Dr. Carol Ann Sperling, a clinical psychologist and director of the Cancer Counseling Institute in Bethesda, Maryland, states that if one gets angry and that particular emotion does not get discharged, and if the resulting hormonal products and small particles such as neurotransmitters and endorphins do not get used, then this in turn cannot benefit the immune system. Dr. Sperling goes further to say that these chemicals sink down, yet they don't go away, and the residue can become toxic in our bodies. It is important to note, however, that immune suppression is a symptom of chronic stress, not short-term stress at normal levels.

Very often when we are feeling sick or weak, I believe that it is nature's way of getting our attention. It is like we have an internal "psychiatrist" who is trying to get our attention to help us make better life decisions. *I truly believe that the condition of fibromyalgia is more directly caused by stress and trauma than any other one thing. If we stop and really think about it, the mind has a much greater influence that we realize.* I can remember times when I was under a great deal of stress and would eventually catch a cold. I can also remember times when I made a commitment that I needed to keep and simply would not allow myself to become sick because I could not "afford" to. I also remember times when I was exposed to a virus or other illnesses that were running rampant, and I would not contract them because of what I believe was a combination of mental determination and a strong immune system.

It seems apparent that we can prevent the onset of disease or lessen the impact of a disease or stimulate the healing of a condition of a disease by adjusting our mental outlook. In traditional medicine, Russian scientists were the first to express this viewpoint—although they were sternly ridiculed in the beginning by some conservative immunologists in the field who argued that immune responses should be observed in the test tube, not the mind. However, in the past ten years, a neurophysiologist, Dr. Novera Herbert Spector, at the National Institute of Health in Bethesda, Maryland, has been conducting research and now suggests that new studies make it very clear that mental attitude can make a significant difference in a person's health. My personal research (based on my clients' health successes) supports Dr. Spector's hypothesis.

Furthermore, a husband/wife radio therapist team, Dr. O. Carl Simonton and Stephanie Simonton, have developed a "whole person approach" to combating disease. The "Simonton Method" calls for the patient to positively alter their emotions, expectations and attitudes in order to fight disease. Daily exercises for relaxation, imaging and physical activity are very important to this process, according to the

Simontons. They verify in their research that an individual's wellness or illness involves not simply the physiology of the body, but rather the whole person—both body and mind. The basic premise behind this theory is that mental therapy uses emotions to prod certain brain chemicals into stimulating the body's defense systems against the invading disease. Endorphins and catecholamines (epinephrine, norepinephrine and dopamine), as well as the T cells from the thymus gland, enhance the immune system's ability to fight disease and assist an individual in getting well.

In response to these theories, a new category for fibromyalgia treatment has been developed called "mind-body therapies." Yoga, biofeedback, meditation, hypnosis, relaxation training and guided imagery are all considered mind-body therapies. Although MBT has met with some criticism, these alternatives offer more options for fibromyalgics suffering from daily pain and fatigue not relieved by traditional medicine. I suggest some relaxation, imaging and positive thinking exercises at the end of this section.

Dr. Norman Cousins

One mind-body theory for fighting illness was introduced by Dr. Norman Cousins in his 1979 book *Anatomy of an Illness* that has sparked recent MBT research. In it, Dr. Cousins describes how he made a miraculous recovery from a long debilitating illness through laughter. Cousins used laughter in a conscious effort to mobilize and enhance his will to live. Dr. Cousins, who was a senior lecturer in medicine at UCLA and a long-time editor of *Saturday Review*, had a disease called ankylosing spondylitis and was told by a specialist that he had a one in 500 chance of recovering from this progressive and incurable disease. Dr. Cousins agreed with the specialist about one thing—if he lingered in a hospital, harassed with taking pain medications and going through x-rays, that indeed certainly would be the case. He checked out of the hospital and proceeded to work with his doctor to devise his own treatment plan. His plan consisted of three parts:

1. He stopped taking all medications, believing that painkillers inhibit the body's self-healing processes.
2. He took megadoses of vitamin C intravenously.
3. And perhaps the most important part, he set out to stop the disease by cultivating the positive emotions of laughter, faith, love, hope and the will to live.

He noted that even ten minutes of genuine, deep laughter before bed would give him at least two hours of deep, restful, pain-free sleep. His healing method was unconventional but miraculously proved to be the most successful, and the once dying Dr. Cousins restored his health and even began playing his two favorite sports—golf and tennis—regularly.

Is Laughter the Best Medicine?

Sparked by the success of Dr. Norman Cousins, many researchers have been studying the effects of laughter on terminal illness. In fact, according to ABC News, researchers at UCLA's Jonsson Cancer Center are prescribing laughter for sick children in hopes that it will boost their immune systems. Although initial studies have focused on healthy children's responses to old comic greats like the Marx Brothers and Abbott & Costello, researchers hope to use their findings to help children undergoing chemotherapy and other somewhat frightening procedures deal with their fear and stress. They hope to prove that laughter not only helps children deal with the immediate pain and fear of illness, but also promotes health and healing.

The Success Attitude

According to Dr. Cousins, attitude is a significant part of our success in fighting disease. Attitude is generally described as our feelings or perception about circumstances, other people, and more importantly, about ourselves. Poor attitude causes more people not to achieve or get to where they want to be with health and finances, and in their families and careers than any other factor.

It is critical for us to understand how our attitude can make us or break us. Our attitude influences our smile, our hand-shake, our appearance, the words we speak, as well as the actions we take or don't take. It is all these things put together that determine whether we will be successful and just how successful we will become—including whether we will get well and stay well.

Because of the vital role of a positive attitude can have in your success, the process outlined for you in this section is vital for your recovery and health. Remember that your body will respond chemically and manifest your thoughts. If you think healthy, positive thoughts, you will begin to create a momentum toward health and vitality. It is true, you can literally choose to be healthy, happy and successful.

Take a moment and think about what your thoughts are about being healthy and completely restored. Do you think these positive thoughts on a consistent basis? Are you thinking only healthy, recovering, alive thoughts or do you focus on the negative as you proceed through each day? Remember that you have a choice. You can expect to get sicker or expect to get well? Are you visualizing health and vitality, happiness and a pain-free body? As John Dorphine said: "The mind is its own place, and in itself can make heaven of hell, or a hell of heaven."

I have decided to include this section in the book because I have an unshakable belief in the power of will, faith and hope for healing all types of problems, whether they be mental or physical, or a combination of the two. For more than fifteen years now, I have done counseling on an individual basis, as well as on a group basis, and many of my clients have benefited greatly from the procedures outlined here. The following four major components are the ingredients for building a positive, successful attitude. When you effectively put the four together (and combine them with the 6-step action plan in Chapter 5), you will possess the means, the attitude and the prowess to get well, be successful and accomplish whatever you choose to do:

- Desire and belief
- Positive self-expectancy
- Visualization
- Preparation for recovery

Desire and Belief

I have chosen to place desire and belief together for an important purpose. These are, in my opinion, the two central ingredients to motivation and achievement. All meaningful achievement and success have their beginnings in desire and are brought to fruition only if one believes strongly enough that it will happen. The most important realization about desire is that it must come from within. You cannot and will not get well or become successful simply because your parents, your spouse, your coach, your supervisor or manager want you to. Even this book, on its own, cannot help you without your own desires and efforts. The answer to every problem or the key to any solution is within you, and your will and desire to succeed must come from within. The more desire you have, the less you limit your potential and the more you will be able to accomplish.

You must truly desire to have your health back. You may say, of course I desire to be healthy again! But it isn't always that simple. The longer you are sick and the more debilitating the illness, the more familiar that state of being becomes. For many, especially those with severe chronic illness, the life changes that accompany a return to health can seem scary. Chronically ill individuals want to be healthy again but may worry about taking on all the responsibilities they had to relinquish because of illness. They may worry that they will relapse or that they won't be able to pick up where they left off. This chapter is included specifically to spark your desire for health, to awaken your hope in your ability to heal and to help you realize your potential for getting well, being happy and becoming successful.

Desire is not effective without the second key, however: belief. Belief (or faith) is an attribute that all positive people exhibit. Nothing of any great significance was ever accomplished without the component of belief—belief in yourself, in others, in life. The basis for belief is confidence and positive thinking. Positive, successful people exude an air of confidence and appear to be in complete control most of the time, despite troubles and failures, because they trust life and themselves. This confidence enables individuals to perform well, even under pressure. In fact, it is usually those without a strong sense of belief and those who lack confidence who generally fall apart under pressure.

Roger Staubach was asked how the Dallas Cowboys always seemed to be successful in coming from behind and winning game after game in the last two minutes. Roger responded, "At the end of every practice, we run a two-minute drill and our goal is to run sixty perfect pass plays. If someone jumps count or drops the ball on the 52nd pass play, for instance, we start back at number one until we run sixty perfect plays. Then in the game, you see, it is second nature for us to run the two-minute drill to perfection. We have instilled such an air of confidence and belief, it's really hard not to accomplish what we set out to do." Once you allow yourself to see the possibility of reversing fibromyalgia, you must expect it and plan for it, believe it can be a reality for you and do everything to can to make your return to health a reality.

Positive Self-Expectancy

It has been said that one of the most outwardly recognizable characteristics of healthy, successful people is positive self-expectancy—that is, they expect positive results in their lives despite disappointments. For example, Bruce Jenner, after having lost every event in the decathlon in Munich, was interviewed in the streets of the Olympic Village. He was asked what he would do now that his Olympic career was over. He replied, "I don't think you understand, I will win the decathlon in Montreal four years from now." With that image of positive self-expectation etched into his subconscious mind, Bruce set out, arising early every day and working persistently toward his goal of becoming the best athlete in the world, and won the decathlon in Montreal.

Research done on the subconscious mind and human performance in the past century has revolutionized our thinking on the power of the mind and human capability. In fact, this research stimulated William James, the renowned psychologist, to state, "The greatest discovery of my lifetime has been that man can alter his life by altering his attitude."

Dr. Joseph Murphy, in his wonderful book, *The Power of Your Subconscious Mind*, explains in detail the psychological power of expectancy. For instance, he explains the "passing-over technique," which consists essentially of inducing the subconscious mind to take over your request of what you want to happen as given it by the conscious mind. Dr. Murphy explains that this "passing over" is best accomplished in a reverie-like state (i.e. a very quiet, relaxed state). This way, the kinetic energy of the subconscious produces positive, successful, pleasant thoughts. Dr. Murphy says, "Just know that in your deeper mind is Infinite Intelligence and Infinite Power, so calmly structure in your mind what you want to happen and vividly imagine it coming into fruition from that moment on."

The power of positive self-expectation has been realized and recognized by mankind throughout the ages. Wise King

Solomon in the 8th century B.C. stated, "As a man thinketh in his heart, so is he." Centuries later, Marcus Aurelius, the Roman emperor and philosopher, wrote "A man's life is what his thoughts make of it." And in his research, Dr. Denis Waitley has reinforced that "we will tend to perform the way we see ourselves in our mind's eye." Finally, Earl Nightingale, after a lifetime of research and study of human nature, was prompted to quote Emerson and conclude, "You will become what you think about all day long."

The power of expectation is both intrinsic and extrinsic. In other words, we not only respond and move toward our own expectations but, at the same time, we are impacted by the expectations of others for us. Our parents, spouses, teachers, supervisors, coaches and peers have a marked influence on our efforts and accomplishments. A combination of expectations from those in our circle of influence and our own belief in our-selves is the key to our success—or our failure. So then, isn't it quite exciting to contemplate the fact that each of us has with-in us the built-in mechanism to utilize positive self-expectancy to get well, be happy and become successful?

Visualization

As mentioned, expecting the positive involves thinking posi-tive thoughts. Visualization is a great way to practice thinking positive and is nothing more than mental imaging. All success-ful people have mastered the art of mental imaging and prac-tice some form of visualization on a consistent basis. You can literally control your destiny by etching in your mind the images of the things you want. The mind is an amazing mech-anism that functions like a heat-seeking missile—the images that we hold consistently in the mind, we will move toward and bring into reality. We can become only what we believe we already are.

An example of this phenomenon in action is evidenced in an amazing story about a United States Air Force officer from

Oregon who was captured and spent seven years in a Vietnamese prisoner-of-war camp. Before his capture he had been a par golfer. Approximately six weeks after his release, he was invited to play in the New Orleans Professional/Amateur Tournament and shot a seventy-six—only four strokes over par. A reporter interviewed him and remarked that his feat was quite phenomenal since he had not touched a golf club in seven years. He explained that it was not a phenomenal feat at all because he had played eighteen holes of golf in his mind every day for seven years. He explained that he visualized the course precisely, saw every fairway, bunker and green vividly in his mind. He studied every shot, selected every club very carefully and would imagine each swing whether it was a drive, chip or putt with perfect technique.

Although you may not be in a prison camp, suffering with fibromyalgia can feel like a prison because it limits what you can do physically. Visualization can help you as it did the Air Force officer from Oregon. Develop the habit of visualizing at various times—while showering and dressing in the morning, when sitting at your desk, before a meeting, during exercise, or while listening to motivational tapes. Picture yourself consistently as a healthy, vibrant individual enjoying the things that give you purpose, choice and passion. Visualization will help you develop confidence and help remove doubt and fear. This feeling of confidence, combined with the visualization, enhances your positive attitude and promotes success and wellness.

Preparation for Recovery

Successful people are made, not born. The reason people are successful is definitely not education or talent alone. There are thousands of educated derelicts, as well as thousands of people with great raw talent who have never accomplished anything above the average or mediocre.

The first thing to accept and understand is that you reach your goals and desired destinations through commitment, persistence, belief and hard work, whether it is a change in careers or reversing chronic illness. Sales leaders spend hours daily on self-improvement, planning and organizational skills. Colonel Sanders was told "no" 1,009 times before receiving a "yes" on his chicken recipe that eventually led to his success. "Pistol Pete" Maravich, an All-American basketball player at LSU, averaged an amazing 44.8 points per game for his collegiate career. His scoring average still stands as a NCAA record after more than twenty years. Every day Pete would arrive at practice an hour or two before the regular practice time to work on his conditioning, shooting skills and ball-handling skills. He became the best through practice, practice, practice—not simply by being born talented. In all successful people you will discover a positive attitude. And within the positive attitude you will always find the ingredients of desire and belief, positive self-expectancy and the ability to visualize success. They also all have a willingness to persevere as they prepare and expect to move toward their desired goal. Preparing for success means not only thinking positively, but also coming up with a specific plan for change. The rest of this chapter is set up to help you plan your fibromyalgia reversal, and success with your family, in your social life and with your business or other endeavors.

Positive Beginnings

One of the best ways to integrate these concepts is to develop a positive-habit pattern. Perhaps one of the most important steps is the first one—awaken each day with a thankful heart and a positive, optimistic attitude with which to program the subconscious mind for total success throughout the day. Remember, as you first begin to gain consciousness in the early morning, the brain is functioning at the subconscious or alpha level and there are only ten to twelve brain wave lengths per second. Therefore, whatever you program at this point or allow to be etched on the subconscious will go with you throughout

"You wrote everything I wanted to say!"

I just finished reading your book *Reversing Fibromyalgia* and wanted to let you know I thought it was fantastic! I have been a fibromyalgia sufferer for thirteen years. After a seven-year exhausting and expensive search to find a diagnosis, I started another exhausting search to find the cure. In February of 1998, a friend introduced me to a company that sells supplemental nutrients. Within one month the quality of my daily life was returning.

I had refused to read any more books about fibromyalgia because I felt no one was really giving us any answers or hope. A friend recommended I read your book. I found I could not put it down! Every supplement you recommend we needed was already in these products I was taking. But I truly loved how you included the spiritual and positive thinking chapter. That was so important to me. I know after my thirteen-year battle I had lost hope, faith and was definitely a negative thinker.

After rebuilding my body, I'm rebuilding my mind and my soul. After feeling better I started going to a personal trainer every day. We slowly stretched my muscles (the very ones you have in your book) and started rebuilding my muscles with the elastic rope as you mentioned. In the beginning, it was very difficult and painful, but as time went on, I became a new person. Every morning I had to do just as you said, think positive thoughts and tell myself I could do this.

When someone asks me to explain my disorder I tell them that I started seeing everything in gray. There was no color in my life, but the worse part for me was losing my smile. I now see the blue sky, the green trees, the beautiful flowers in bloom, and I can't wait for the beautiful fall colors that will be coming, and my husband says I even smile in my sleep now.

I now talk to fibromyalgia sufferers every day. Most of the ones I talk to are already on morphine, Prozac or the many other drugs. Sometimes it is hard to get through to them, but now with the help of your book, maybe they will listen.

I used to ask "why me?" I now know that I needed to let others know that there is hope and your book will be a part of that from now on. They need to know that they can reverse fibromyalgia, not just learn to cope with the pain.

Thank you for taking the time and passion to find out what could possibly be causing this terrible disorder. I feel as if you wrote everything that I wanted to say. Keep up the great work!

Sincerely,

Gina L.

Georgia

the day. This is the point daily at which you decide whether you will be well, happy, optimistic, productive, successful, etc. Take the following prescription for a positive, uplifting, joyous, rewarding, productive day—every day!

Early Morning

- Awaken early with a thankful heart.
- Visualize yourself as a winner.
- Read inspirational texts.
- Review your goals.
- Brainstorm ways to improve health and happiness.
- Engage in a brief walk or other exercise daily.
- Shower and prepare the mind.
- Eat a healthy breakfast.

Course of the Day

- Think positive, wholesome thoughts.
- Give a pleasant greeting and smile to everyone.
- Answer greetings with "wonderful" and "fantastic."
- Offer sincere appreciation.
- Listen more, talk less.

- Work with your plan/schedule.
- Be flexible.
- Exercise, play and relax.
- See your work as pleasure.
- Eat a moderate lunch and a reasonable, balanced dinner.
- Allow for family time.

Late Evening

- Keep a success journal.
- Have a thankful heart/review your goals.
- Reflect on today's success.
- Read an inspirational text or listen to relaxing music.
- Plan for tomorrow.
- Brainstorms ideas and solutions for upcoming problems.

Keys for Success

A lifetime of experience, coupled with twenty-five years of research, has yielded the answer to a question that intrigued me for the better part of my life: "Why do some achieve in such an extraordinary fashion, others fail so miserably, and the masses settle for the average or mediocre?" I discovered that many scholars and researchers have sought to answer the same question and have all come to the same basic conclusion: there are common denominators that bring about extraordinary human achievement. The common denominators yielded by my experiences and research are listed below as the "Keys For Success."

Each of the keys or concepts will be explained briefly on the subsequent pages. If you will embrace these principles and concepts and apply them, your chances for reversing fibromyalgia and achieving health and success in all other areas will be enhanced tremendously:

- Establish your values.
- Discover your life purpose.
- Mold a mission.
- Set and write down your goals.
- Come up with an action plan.
- Visualize yourself as a winner.
- Expect the extraordinary.
- Understand motivation.
- Learn to communicate.
- Have a thankful heart.
- Become a serious student.
- Discover the magic of giving.

Establish Your Values

To succeed at any goal, a person must identify and understand what is most important to them, what they value most, and what they would fight for and defend. Until individuals establish this baseline, it is impossible to set meaningful goals and choose direction in life.

Discover Your Life Purpose

Once you know what is most important to you, it will be easier for you to discover what your purpose in life is. Every individual possesses specific and unique gifts and talents to carry out a particular purpose in this life. In other words, every life has a purpose and will achieve total peace and contentment only if they are working and serving within their particular purpose. Engage your family members, friends, work associates, teammates, etc. to assist you in affirming your gifts and talents. This one thing will assist you more than any other in determining your life purpose. This and other techniques will be presented later to assist you in making your purpose decisions in life (i.e., going on vacation, the promotion to vice-president, which civic club to join, going out for the team, taking a computer course, and choosing your college major, your life vocation, or the person to marry). Knowing your life purpose will also help give you the hope and drive to get better.

Mold a Mission

Once your values are established and you have a feel for the talents and abilities that clue you in to your life purpose, you can begin to mold a mission. It does not occur to many people that they were given special gifts and traits that they can excel in. You were given the wherewithal to carve out your niche in life, so follow these steps and go for it.

Many never realize their potential and never accomplish their purpose because they never received the knowledge and facts presented to you now. Most go to school for twelve to twenty years and never have a course that teaches them what to do with their knowledge. Once you realize your life has a purpose and once you begin to move toward something you really desire, life gets exciting and you can begin to mold a mission (set life goals) that will get you up each morning with enthusiasm and will ultimately stimulate the production of life-sustaining and healing hormones.

Set and Write Down Your Goals

One major mistake that many people make is that they attempt to set goals before establishing their values and understanding their purpose for existing. It is only after we do these things that establishing goals carries a magic that etches them indelibly into our subconscious mind. Research has proven this important concept time and again: the images we hold constantly in our mind will eventually come to pass.

Ralph Waldo Emerson was referring to the immeasurable human potential when he wrote, "What lies before us and what lies behind us pales in significance when we realize what lies within us." The goal setting principles in this chapter are meant to help you realize the vast potential within. Once we begin to set goals, visions begin to be etched on the subconscious mind. As these visions become crystallized in our mind's eye, we begin to get excited about life and generate an enthusiasm that eventually results in action that transforms our dreams into reality. As we move toward accomplishment and begin to feel the exhilaration of the fulfillment of all that we were intended to be, we begin to experience the abundance and inner peace that has been promised in life.

Guidelines for Goal Setting

Principle One: Things won't change until you change. Make the commitment now to develop healthier habits. Consistent, productive, positive habits will lead to goal achievement and success. Successful people are not those without problems, they simply learn to be persistent and are willing to solve their problems.

Principle Two: The goal-setting process is tedious and time consuming. Make the commitment now to invest ample time for planning and structuring your life for success. Commit to developing new habits to support your time investment (i.e., reviewing and revising your goals frequently, arising early, being prompt, returning calls, completing assignments, develop a thankful attitude rather than a critical one).

Principle Three: You won't get much by demand; it's what you do by performance that will yield results. It comes from within you; you have all the answers, gifts, talents within you to achieve your goals and your desires.

Principle Four: Don't wish it were easier, wish you were better. Remember that your obstacles, crises and setbacks are your greatest assets. It is through overcoming these that you become stronger, wiser, better. Emerson said, "When man sits on the cushions of comfort he goes to sleep, but when he sits on the needles of adversity he rises up to do great things."

Principle Five: It is not what happens to you, it's how you respond to what happens that makes the difference in success and failure. Your experiences plus your responses have determined where you are, who you are and what you are.

Principle Six: Life is not a destination, it's a journey. The key to fulfillment in life is to realize that it's not what you get at the end that's important, but what you become in the process. Cervantes summed it up when he stated, "The road is much better than the end."

Come Up with an Action Plan

It has been written that the best plan in the world will not work if you won't. Without a plan of action, a goal remains in the dream category and will eventually fade away. *Remember that motivation and positive feelings come after taking action.* Many are deceived into thinking that one gets motivated, then acts. This principle is illustrated by the fellow sitting before the wood stove and saying, "Give me some heat and I will then put some wood in you." And when you chop your own wood, you warm yourself twice.

These same concepts apply to your goal to reverse fibromyalgia. Once you begin making changes in how you live and see the positive effects your changes have on your health, you will feel more motivated to make further changes. The success your actions bring will give you hope to overcome and a reason to be healthy again. Taking action heals because it gives you a sense that you have some control over your life and how you feel again.

Your action plan will be your daily road map. Could you imagine building a house without the plan? A builder would need to know the specifics of how many square feet, the exact materials, the style of home with every detail, in order to produce the desired home. Your plan should include reachable, concrete goals that you set each day, each week, each month, each year. Establish a long-term goal and break it down into manageable pieces that you can do daily or weekly. For instance, you may want to eat healthier as a long-term goal. If you suddenly gave up your normal diet and adopted a completely foreign one, your chances of success are pretty low. Not only is the task of overhauling everything at once pretty daunting, but maintaining your new habits will be difficult because you are adopting so many at once. Instead, what if you decide to give up one unhealthy eating habit each week (i.e. caffeine) and replace it with a healthier one (i.e. drinking more water)? Within weeks you would have a new diet that you adopted piece by piece, practically stress-free. This book can help you with an action plan for reversing fibromyalgia by giving you ideas for short and long-term goals to improve your health.

Visualize Yourself as a Winner

The success of our goals depends on our belief that they can be accomplished. The most powerful mechanism we have available for success is the ability of the subconscious mind to imagine or visualize what we want to happen. Unfortunately, it works in the negative as well—we can literally destroy ourselves with worry, doubt and fear. Therefore, it is vital to train the subconscious to cancel out the negative and consistently nurture the positive.

Earlier in this chapter you were introduced to a set of early-morning activities meant to train you to develop positive mental habits characteristic of highly successful people. It takes approximately twenty-one days to develop a habit. So as you consistently visualize your success, you will begin to walk, talk and perform successfully in all areas of your life. As you learn to focus on your goals and the person you are becoming, your subconscious mind will attract, like a magnet, the people and resources needed to help you achieve success. As you learn to consistently utilize this gift of visualization, miracles will begin to occur in your life and circumstances.

As you move forward and set goals, don't worry about how these things will come about, simply move forward in faith, keep your visions clear, work hard every day with a sense of purpose and enjoy the miracles as they occur in your life. So start seeing yourself healthy and happy from this point on.

Expect the Extraordinary

"You may not always get what you want, but you will almost always get what you expect." Dr. Denis Waitley recognized that the most outward, recognizable characteristic of a successful person is positive self-expectation. Earl Nightingale stated that winners are never surprised when they win, simply because that was their expectation from the outset. Positive thinking or optimism is an empowering state of mind or attitude that will bring about extraordinary results. Dozens of research studies in psychology and education have proven that we will produce precisely what we expect from ourselves and what others feel we are capable of producing.

As we raise our own self-expectancy and self-image, others will raise their expectations and respect for us. The old adage that our attitude will determine our altitude has certainly been born out. Psychologists have proven through research that the 80 percent of the total population that do not perform up to their capability typically have a poor self-image and low expectations. The major difference between those 80 percent and the 20 percent of successful people is simply attitude. It is vital, then, to expect the extraordinary from ourselves.

Every human being is unique and possesses the gifts and talents to be extraordinary at something—the key is to seek that special purpose in life and then be expectant of the extraordinary, and it will most assuredly happen. Dr. Norman Vincent Peale sums it up in his classic book, *The Power of Positive Thinking*, when he concludes, "If you think positive thoughts, you purely and simply will get positive results."

Understand Motivation

Learning the art of motivation is one of the critical keys to success. One of the most empowering factors for motivation in goal setting is to list the reasons for desiring to achieve each goal. Remember, without specific reasons for achieving your goals, you are much less likely to accomplish them. When we learn to utilize and respond positively to feedback, we will employ the art of motivation. Two kinds of feedback provide awareness and empowerment that move us toward our life goals.

The first, internal feedback is the inner emotional feeling or response we feel as we perceive an action, a thought or a circumstance. This inner response can come from our own thought and actions, successes or failures, or from the observation of statements, actions or circumstances of others. These feelings and perceptions can range anywhere from exhilaration to depression to any place in between. Whether positive or negative, we can learn from this internal feedback, take the invaluable data, program it into our library of information and utilize it for future reference, either to avoid the pitfalls of failure or for the accomplishment of successes.

The second, external feedback, comes from others through direct responses, acceptance, rejection, opinions, evaluations, constructive criticisms, etc. Once again, whether positive or negative, it can be invaluable in moving us toward our successes while assisting us in avoiding pitfalls.

Learn to Communicate

Every successful person considers himself or herself an ongoing self-improvement project. A major part of this self-improvement is the art of communication. Those who master it in this high-tech world will have access to success and the universe. The wise and successful individual will master the skills of listening, speaking and writing. The ability to watch, read, hear and interpret the thoughts, ideas, needs and desires of others is critical in the processes and procedures of success. Equally important is developing the ability to convey your thoughts, ideas, needs and desires to others effectively.

Have a Thankful Heart

Developing an attitude of gratitude is one of the most powerful things you can do in your life to bring about positive changes that will bring success and generate feelings of peace, contentment and enthusiasm. When you express gratitude for all parts of your life daily, you begin to see your life and self in a different, very positive perspective. When you become more thankful for what you have and what has happened, you will begin to excitedly look forward to the future and what will happen.

Become a Serious Student

Knowledge is power. Successful people are very much aware of this basic truth. So, if you are really serious about success, then become a serious student and begin to tap the treasury of knowledge, if you have not already done so. Go to the library, read books, listen to tapes, go to classes, attend the seminars, get on the internet. This book is only the beginning.

Discover the Magic of Giving

Mankind has forever searched for purpose and the reason for existing. The most frequent conclusion reached for man's existence is that we are here to build up, encourage and serve our fellow man. Those who have discovered and employed this secret to life have achieved man's most desired commodity: inner peace.

When we serve, we simply give. Giving is one of the magical keys to success and life. Giving causes us to grow and achieve a maturity and wholeness that can be achieved in no other way. It has been proven time and again that we can only receive back that which we give away. Giving to others has a powerful built-in healing ability.

Further Mind-Body Reading

I would like to recommend some books in the area of the mind-body connection and the role it can play in effectively regaining optimal health:

- *The Healer Within*, by Stephen Locke, M.D. Dr. Locke gives a thorough view of the science of psychoneuroimmunology that is very detailed, but is readable and easy to understand. This book also includes a lengthy appendix of organizations and resources to turn to for further help.
- *Nutrition and Your Immune System*, by Carlson Wade. This book gives you a good understanding of your immune system including definitions, how it works and discussion of the diseases that are caused by a weakened immune system.
- *Love, Medicine, and Miracles*, by Berney S. Siegel, M.D. This is another excellent book in which Dr. Siegel explores the common physiological characteristics of his patients who have recovered from serious illnesses such as cancer.

- *The Success Journal*, by Dr. Joe M. Elrod. My complete success system developed to assist you in achieving your life goals. It contains a life balance scale and a daily, weekly, monthly success tracking system. Refer to the Resource List at the end of this book for information on how to order a copy.

Personal Commitment Statement

Acknowledging that only I can define success for myself, I, _____, agree that my success plan can be designed only by me and fulfilled by my consistent, determined actions. I agree that commitment to my plan is the first step in achieving the success that I desire. I will use this plan to set my goals, and I will use this plan to track my success.

I recognize that to reach my goals and to realize my fullest potential, I must strive consistently with a positive mental attitude. I promise to daily work at improving my skills and increasing my knowledge so as to achieve the realization of getting well and becoming all that I was intended to be. Finally, I will commit to following this plan.

_____   _____

Date   *Signature*

5

Reversing Fibromyalgia: The 6-Step Action Plan

"When written in Chinese, the word 'crisis' is composed of two characters—one represents danger, and the other represents opportunity." – JOHN F. KENNEDY

Now that you have committed to reversing fibromyalgia, let's talk about the specifics of my plan and how it can work for you. I've already mentioned a number of options for treatment—both traditional and alternative—that can do absolutely wonderful things for your fibromyalgia symptoms. However, they are only part of the fibromyalgia cure. The majority of fibromyalgia sufferers I have worked with experienced a traumatic emotional experience, usually of a very long duration, before developing the syndrome. In addition, most of them were not exercising properly, were not eating right, and therefore, did not ingest the proper vitamins, minerals and nutrients. Furthermore, many did not have very good skills for coping with stress. As a result, their immune systems began to break down over time, and they began to experience fibromyalgia symptoms.

In response to these problems, I developed a six-step action plan that I have successfully used for over ten years in my

Figure 3. A reversal model for fibromyalgia

1. Return to Restful Sleep
2. Detoxify and Cleanse the Body
3. Use Nutritional Supplements
4. Adopt a Healthy Nutrition Program
5. Adhere to an Exercise Program
6. Develop Stress Management Skills

research. This plan (shown in figure 3) has helped dozens of fibromyalgia sufferers reverse their symptoms and begin on a trek to restored health and vitality. The steps are designed to work synergistically (all together) to rebuild an impaired immune system. When the immune system is restored, the body can regenerate cells and heal itself. Although this series of steps is not a cure-all and will not work 100 percent for everyone, I believe it is the most complete and effective regimen for reversing fibromyalgia to date. Additionally, because of its natural emphasis, the potential for side effects is almost nonexistent.

Consult Your Physician or a Health Professional

As mentioned earlier, since there are many physical conditions that are very similar to or coincide with fibromyalgia, the symptoms can be very confusing or misleading to the patient (and sometimes the physician). Because of the complexity of fibromyalgia, it is important that you do not rely on self-diagnosis and self-treatment. With fibromyalgia or any other chronic condition, it is vitally important to get a correct diagnosis and prescription for treatment. For example, I was recently conducting a seminar in Atlanta and was approached by a couple who inquired about fibromyalgia symptoms. I was informed that the husband was suffering with fibromyalgia. I talked with them for some time, asked many of the questions I normally ask, and then did some diagnosis by palpation. I discovered that the gentleman had pain only on one area of his body. He did not have fibromyalgia, but instead had a problem with his rotator cuff in the right shoulder. He needed to get help from an orthopedic specialist for proper diagnosis and treatment.

If you suspect fibromyalgia, be certain to get a thorough evaluation and have a consultation with at least one medical doctor, preferably a rheumatologist who has experience with the condition. Even if you are reasonably certain that you have fibromyalgia, *be sure to consult with your physician and have an examination before starting this program.*

Dr. Elrod's 6-Step Action Plan

Step #1: Return to Restful Sleep

As mentioned in the first chapter, sleeping disorders are probably one of the most devastating symptoms associated with fibromyalgia. Pain in the muscles and connective tissues makes deep sleep almost impossible, and sleep disruptions interfere with the production of growth hormone needed for healthy muscles and soft tissue. Most fibromyalgia patients do not get enough rest—even after eight hours of sleep.

Deep sleep (level 4) allows the body to replenish itself and helps defend against chronic fatigue, stress and depression. Without it, our immune systems are weakened, and we are more susceptible to chronic illnesses like fibromyalgia. Because a lack of deep sleep is intimately linked with the development and perpetuation of fibromyalgia symptoms, restful sleep is one of the keys to restoring your health and returning to an active, vibrant lifestyle.

Most fibromyalgia sufferers will have difficulty sleeping, either awakening several times during the night or engaging in light sleep, and generally will wake up feeling very tired. In a research study done within a sleep lab, researchers found that fibromyalgia patients could fall asleep without much difficulty because of fatigue; however, their deep sleep level was constantly interrupted by bursts of "awake-like" brain activity. Many fibromyalgia patients have an associated deep sleep disorder called the "alpha-EEG anomaly" (Hauri, 1973). They appear to spend the night in and out of light sleep, awakening in the early morning with an unrefreshed feeling.

As a result of sleeplessness and fatigue, most fibromyalgia patients feel totally drained of energy. The fatigue symptom can be mild in some and incapacitating in others, but 90 percent of the patients with fibromyalgia describe moderate to severe fatigue similar to the exhaustion experienced with the flu. Frequently, the fatigue is more of a problem than the pain. Most of them are unaware that their fatigue is a result of never entering the stage four sleep that is so necessary for health and vitality. Your potential for returning to deep, replenishing sleep is greatly enhanced if you utilize the following suggestions:

- *Stick to a regular exercise program.* Exercise is the most effective way to counteract the effects of stress and is essential for reducing tension. Exercise will strengthen and restore flexibility to your muscles, eventually reducing and eliminating the pain associated with fibromyalgia, and it stimulates the production of growth hormone needed for healthy muscle and soft tissue. Exercise also stimulates the production of T cells to boost the immune system and releases healing, uplifting endorphins that have an antidepressant effect. The combined effects of exercise will also help you sleep better. But remember not to exercise too late in the day, as this could disrupt your sleep.

- *Develop and use good stress management skills.* Take mini-breaks during the day and practice deep breathing and muscle relaxation exercises. Also, take fifteen minutes periodically during the day to do some stretching exercises. These will

"I love your approach"

I am a research scientist here in Utah. Our research and development group purchased your book *Reversing Fibromyalgia,* as many of our customers in the field suffer from this condition.

I just wanted to write you a short note and tell you how much I love your book. I'm reading it for myself, to utilize your advice, even though I'm as healthy as a horse. I love your approach, combining the mind and body, to heal itself. The chapters on exercise, nutrition, and natural supplements and herbal remedies are wonderful too. I am recommending this book to customers that have problems even related to the diseases you address. But I've also recommended it to friends and coworkers, as a good book about life management.

Thanks again for such a marvelous book!

Sincerely,

Camille M.

Utah

increase blood flow, refresh and energize you. I will discuss some of these skills later in the book, but don't be afraid to do some research on your own to find the exercises or activities that will work best for you. Anything that relieves stress can be added to your routine.

- *Take time to play.* Make sure you have enough fun and pleasure in your life. Go on a picnic with your family, take your dog for a walk, write in a journal or go to a movie—whatever it is that you enjoy! Relaxation and good times are therapeutic and rewarding.

- *Cut down on (or cut out) caffeine and alcohol,* especially late in the afternoon and evening. Having a nightcap before going to bed may feel like it is helping initially, but it will actually leave you tired and listless the next morning.

- *Spend the last hour before bed winding down.* Take a relaxing hot bath, review your goals, focus on everything that's joyful, good, happy and positive, or read from stimulating and motivating sources. Establishing a night routine will help prepare your body and your mind for sleep and will empty you of the day's stresses.

- *Follow a healthy nutrition program and supplementation regimen.* Some simple guidelines such as lowering saturated fat, limiting fried foods, increasing fiber and modifying sugar intake will enhance better sleep. Also, eating more fruits and vegetables—along with taking a healthy regimen of vitamins and minerals—tends to have a cleansing and balancing effect on the body that works to promote better sleep. I will discuss diet and nutrient supplementation in more detail later in the book.

- *Develop a regular schedule.* For most people, it helps to develop a routine of retiring and rising at about the same times on a daily basis. It can be devastating for the fibromyalgia sufferer to retire later than normal and miss one good night's sleep. Some of the symptoms may return almost immediately with such a disruption. It may also be a good idea to have meals on regular schedule as well.

- *Try the adaptogenic herb ginseng.* More than four thousand years ago, the Chinese used this herb to tranquilize the spirit, calm agitation of the mind and ward off harmful influences while restoring and revitalizing the internal organs. Adaptogens, essential to plant and animal life, must adapt to changing temperatures, light patterns, and a variety of other stresses.

  Research in Europe and Japan has confirmed ginseng's ability to reduce stress and improve mental function. The most common forms of ginseng are Korean, Chinese and Siberian. Each type works a little differently, so take as directed on the label. Choose a product with a high percentage of ginsenosides, the active ingredients (Tenney, 1995).

• *Try herbal sleeping remedies.* Thirty minutes before retiring, drink one cup of chamomile tea and take two to six milligrams of melatonin. Melatonin is produced by the pineal gland embedded behind your eyes in the brain. As it gets dark, this small gland secretes melatonin to calm, relax and promote sleep. (Experiment with different amounts until you find what's right for you.) Valerian and passionflower also promote relaxation and sleep. For additional advice on natural remedies for sleeping disorders, refer to Chapter 12 of Rita Elkin's *Solving the Depression Puzzle.*

• *Sleep in a comfortable, cool, quiet environment.* Wakefulness and sleeping are regulated by circadian rhythms in a twenty-four hour cycle. This cycle is controlled by exposure to light and the secretion of hormones, particularly melatonin. Utilize heavy curtains to block out light and use music, white noise or recorded nature sounds (e.g. waves or waterfalls) to block outside distracting noises. Also, do not study, work or do other daytime activities in your bedroom.

Step #2: Detoxify and Cleanse the Body

Because of a combination of environmental pollution and the flaws of a modern diet, it is important that everyone, not just those with fibromyalgia, regularly detoxify and cleanse their bodies. The total cleansing process includes blood, digestive tract, colon and total body cleansing. The key is to utilize healthful nutrition and natural nutrient supplementation to thoroughly cleanse the body, removing harmful toxins so that the immune system is boosted and fully functioning for its health restoring and maintenance process.

Building immunity is one of the most essential parts of reversing fibromyalgia. Poor immune function not only makes your body more vulnerable to illness and infection, but also increases your risk for depression, severe fatigue and other health problems. Not only is a weakened immune system the primary problem with systemic conditions such as fibromyalgia, it can also be linked to many secondary conditions that occur with fibromyalgia, like yeast or sinus infections and gastrointestinal disturbances.

Ideally, immune boosting is a year-round endeavor, but it is never too late to start. Even if your immune system is below optimal levels now, with a little work, you can see major improvements after a few weeks. It is not a simple process however—the immune system is influenced by the health and function of the entire body, as well as by outside influences like stress, poor diet, free radical exposure, medications, fatigue and nutrient deficiencies. Because of the complexity of the immune system, "quick fix" immune boosts will have little effect without long-term lifestyle changes like a healthy nutrition and exercise program, stress management techniques and nutrient supplementation. Detoxification is a good first step, however.

The following are suggested supplements to aid you in your detoxification and cleansing program:

- *Red clover.* This herb is a natural blood purifier and builder, most potent in its liquid form. It has been used to give the body strength and energy it needs to protect and strengthen the immune system—especially important for those with fibromyalgia. Some of the better red clover products will have some supplemental herbs added such as echinacea, licorice root, cascara bark and rosemary. It is recommended to take one teaspoon twice daily with a large glass of water or fruit juice.

- *Pau d' arco.* This agent is a natural blood cleanser and builder, and has antibiotic properties to fight infections in the body. It also helps combat cancer and has been used to strengthen the immune system.

- *Apple cider vinegar.* This is one of the best body purifiers and cleansers, especially when used in its organic form. It is usually a very potent formula and is best used when mixed with a healthy juice or purified water. Recommended dosage is one tablespoon twice a day.

- *Acidophilus.* This is a digestive tract and colon cleanser used to replace good bacteria in the digestive tract and to fight disease and infection. Cultured yogurt (with live cultures) is an excellent source of acidophilus.

- *Goldenseal.* Goldenseal assists in boosting a sluggish glandular system and promotes hormonal production. It goes directly into the bloodstream and also assists in regulating liver function. Goldenseal is reported to act as a natural insulin by providing the body with nutrients necessary to produce its own insulin. This aids metabolism and energy production and makes goldenseal a most effective supplement for fibromyalgia. It also acts as a natural antibiotic to stop infections and kill poisons in the body.

- *Magnesium and malic acid.* Make certain that you use a combination of magnesium and malic acid in your healing regimen. This combination is the key to restoring the efficiency of the energy production process that physiologically stimulates the healing process. Malic acid is a food supplement found in citrus fruits and is very plentiful in apples. Some studies have found that it assists energy, metabolism, muscle health, and is most helpful in fibromyalgia. Take as recommended.

See my 21-day detoxification program in Chapter 7 for more information.

Step #3: Use Nutritional Supplements

Authorities now agree that the average American diet no longer provides the needed nutrition for good health. Coffee, white bread, and sugar are the most popular and most often consumed foods. Half of all foods eaten in America are over-processed and convenience foods have little, if any, nutritional value. In fact, 80 percent of middle class American children and 90 percent of American adults are severely malnourished. Both children and adults choose to eat for taste, cost and convenience instead of health. Ironically, most of our pets eat a far better and more nutritionally rich diet than do most American children or adults (Carper, 1995).

Good nutrition provides the antioxidants, bioflavonoids and phytonutrients needed for health and vitality. Antioxidants are known for their special role as a preventative aid in controlling excess oxidation and free radical damage. Free radicals are unstable molecules produced from oxygen and fats. Antioxidants are necessary nutrients and enzymes that buffer or break down free radicals to prevent them from damaging healthy cells (Tenney, 1995). Research has pointed out that polyunsaturated fats are easily converted into free radicals. Oily salad dressings, fried foods and junk foods contain high amounts of polyunsaturated. Most researchers believe that the aging process, some forms of heart disease, cancer, diabetes, and yes, even fibromyalgia are related to free radical damage in the cells.

Highly refined and processed foods contain pollutants and chemical toxins. Fruits and vegetables, unless grown organically, will receive pesticide treatment and be exposed to even more toxins. The water we use, as well as the air we breathe, contains pollutants. Meats are often treated with antibiotics and hormones. These are all reasons why we need nutritional supplementation. Nutrients boost the antioxidant defense system and help protect the body from these environmental pollutants and toxins. The following are some very powerful immune boosters that will assist with your return to health and vitality when combined with other elements of the reversing fibromyalgia program:

- *Bee pollen.* Bee pollen is very high in protein and is considered one of the most complete foods that we can consume. It contains rich sources of vitamins, minerals, amino acids, proteins, enzymes and essential fatty acids. Bee pollen aids hormone imbalances and is very useful to the fibromyalgia patient because it helps to improve the appetite, normalize intestinal activity, strengthen capillary walls, and offset the effects of drugs and pollutants. Bee pollen is also effective for healing colitis and improving anemia. A very high grade of bee pollen, preferably in granular form, should be sought out and can generally be found in health food stores. Those with allergies may need to start with as little as one granule per day in order to build up a tolerance to any allergic reaction. Suggested dosage is one teaspoon of granules per day.

- *B vitamins.* Vitamin B12 is central to immune processes and deficiencies of vitamin B6 lower white blood cell count and shrink the thymus.

- *Coenzyme Q10.* This is a powerful antioxidant that increases circulation and is used by the muscles for energy and to enhance metabolism. Co Q10 is believed to be about twenty times stronger than vitamin E. Suggested dosage is 50 mg minimum per day.

- *Echinacea.* Echinacea is a powerful herb that stimulates immune response and helps the body increase its ability to resist infection, produce white blood cells and purify the blood. Echinacea is considered to be a natural antibiotic.

- *Iron, chromium and manganese.* A deficiency of iron paralyzes the immune system, and excess iron also hurts immunity.

Chromium enhances the effectiveness of white blood cells, and manganese boosts NK cell activity.

- *Pycnogenol (proanthocyanidin).* This is a very powerful antioxidant extracted from grape seed or pine bark. According to researchers, grape seed extract appears to be a potent immune booster and is an antioxidant fifty times stronger than vitamin E. Pycnogenol strengthens collagen (the reinforcement bars of the cells), improves circulation, and enhances the permeability of cell walls. It enhances metabolism and promotes a healing effect in the body. Suggested dosage is 50–200 mg daily, depending upon the severity of the condition.

- *Rice bran extract.* There are three polyphenols from the tocotryonols of rice bran that are 6,000 times stronger than vitamin E.

- *Selenium and zinc.* These two trace minerals are very powerful antioxidants and are essential to boosting the immune system and the healing process. Selenium works synergistically with other nutrients, especially vitamin E. It assists the body in utilizing oxygen and helps with normal growth function and healing. Two good sources of selenium are alfalfa and kelp. Zinc helps with the absorption of vitamins in the body and assists in the formation of skin, hair and nails. It is an essential part of many enzymes involved in digestion, metabolism and the creation of energy. Zinc is also essential to the growth process. Ginseng and kelp are good sources of zinc. Vitamin A must be present for zinc to be properly absorbed by the body. Recommended dosage for selenium is 250 micrograms per day and for zinc 30 milligrams per day. More than 100 mg of zinc per day is immunosuppressive.

- *Vitamins A, C and E.* All three vitamins have antioxidant functions. Vitamin A enhances white blood cell function and the body's resistance to infection. Vitamin A is often used in conjunction with zinc. Vitamin C is a staple item in any immune boosting program and is the ultimate immune booster. Vitamin E fights infection, but large doses may suppress the immune system.

(See the Resource Guide for more information on immune boosters.)

Step #4: Adopt a Healthy Nutrition Program

Nutrition is also important for building immunity because the immune system is responds to the slightest changes in the balance of nutrients in the body. And as mentioned, nutrition is a critical factor in the treatment and healing of fibromyalgia. A healthy diet will not only enhance your chances of recovering from fibromyalgia, it will also protect you against cancer, heart disease, arthritis, diabetes and stroke. For the body to recover and function at peak performance, you need a proper balance of a wide variety of foods including complex carbohydrates, helpful fats, protein, fiber, vitamins, minerals, phytochemicals and potent bioflavonoids.

Furthermore, eating healthy doesn't just involve the types of food you eat, but other eating habits and practices. It may mean eating five or six small meals daily; boiling, broiling, baking and steaming while limiting fried foods; and never skipping meals, especially breakfast. Chapters 6, 7 and 8 provide a more complete nutritional and supplemental guide for reversing fibromyalgia.

Step #5: Adhere to an Exercise Program

Exercise is one of the best methods for preventing obesity, chronic illnesses (like heart disease and diabetes) and depression. Exercise improves muscle tone as it increases blood flow into the tissues. It also increases flexibility and range of motion, stimulates the production of healing endorphins, and enhances T cells to boost immune function. Exercise also stimulates serotonin and growth hormone production.

For those with fibromyalgia, the right exercises are essential to weight control and improved sleep as well as pain reduction and increased mobility. Another outstanding benefit of exercise to the fibromyalgia patient is the improved health of the supportive structures and joints. At one time, it was thought that exercise actually caused arthritis; however, we now know regular exercise is an excellent means of helping to keep joints healthy. For more information on exercise and fibromyalgia see Chapter 9.

(See the Resource Guide for more information on the Body Advantage exercise system.)

Step #6: Develop Stress Management Skills

Effective techniques for dealing with stress can assist fibromyalgia patients in fighting stress and depression. Stress is the response of the mind, body and emotions to everyday happenings and the pressures of life. It is important to recognize that stress is not the actual event, but rather our interpretation of and emotional reaction to the event. For example, a very active person might find a stress fracture injury very traumatic while the next person may find it an opportunity to rest up and refresh the body while recovering. The event (injury) is the same, but the perception of the event by the two people is different and so the response is different. It is individual response that determines the stress impact (O'Koon, 1996). And the impact of stress on the body is very real.

Recent studies on chronic stress link it to problems like memory impairment, flu, poor wound healing, adult-onset diabetes, hypertension and heart attacks, cancer and AIDS—to name a few (Meyer, 2000). Doctor Esther Sternberg says in her book, *The Balance Within: The Science Connecting Health and Emotions* (2000), that short-term stress can be beneficial in a situation by boosting your immunity and helping you focus your thoughts and even your vision to help you respond quickly in a stressful situation. Chronic stress, however, floods the body with stress-related hormones and chemicals that debilitate you over time. One of the most deadly affects of chronic stress is suppressed immunity.

Chronic stress can be particularly debilitating to those with fibromyalgia because of its effects on the immune system. It is essential that fibromyalgia sufferers develop stress management skills and build stress buffers in their daily schedules. Paul J. Rosch of the American Institute of Stress (www.stress.org) advises that individuals be flexible with their stress-fighting strategies because no one approach will work for everyone (Meyer, 2000). Below are some guidelines for coping with stress to get you started. For more detailed information refer to Chapter 10.

- *Boost your nutrition by eating more frequently,* four to five times a day, and choosing an abundance of complex carbohydrates and high fiber foods such as whole grains, whole grain breads and cereals, rice, pasta, beans, peas and potatoes, along with plenty of fresh fruits and vegetables. Only 20 percent of your total food volume should be fat. Avoid sugar, caffeine, and stay away from sugar-laden foods. Ingest a reasonable number of calories to enhance your weight loss and/or weight maintenance program.

- *Vitamin and mineral supplements* of any antioxidant combination will boost the immune system and enhance the cellular cleansing process by maintaining and invigorating cellular energy, cardiovascular awareness, and youthful vitality.

- *Get regular exercise.* Cycle, walk or swim a minimum of four to five times per week for aerobic exercise. Include stretching and muscle toning exercises two to three days per week. Don't overdo it. Even mild activity each day will help your

Janice: A Story of Success

Janice, a 38-year-old, married mother of three, worked very hard as a seventh grade teacher. She was always on the go but felt happy and seemed healthy. Even with work and home responsibilites, she still managed to attend aerobics classes three days a week and take time for herself. Then, one morning when she attempted to get out of bed, she experienced a dull, aching pain in her neck and shoulder region for no apparent reason. At first, the pain only struck in the early morning as she was getting up, but very soon it began to hurt during the day— when standing and teaching in the classroom, sitting at her desk, and finally, even when she was sleeping. There seemed to be no real pattern to the pain, except that it grew steadily worse and seemed to spread to other parts of her body.

Fortunately, Janice had excellent medical insurance and didn't hesitate to make an appointment with her physician. But after an exhaustive testing session, absolutely nothing showed up. Her blood work seemed to be normal, her blood pressure was okay, and nothing was found from tests on specific parts of the body, so she was told by her physician that there seemed to be nothing wrong. She was just advised to take Tylenol for the pain.

After her visit, the pain continued to spread to other parts of her body, and she had more difficulty sleeping. In response, her doctor took her off Tylenol and advised her to take ibuprofen. He eventually told her that he felt there was not much that could be done. Her family didn't really understand the problem either since the medical tests had not found anything.

Janice found herself in a sort of catch-22, where everything she was doing to relieve the pain and frustration of her illness actually was causing her more stress and frustration and further aggravating her mystery symptoms. And so less than two years after the pain and stiffness first appeared, Janice was forced to stop doing many of the things she had previously done for her three small children. Nor did she have the energy or stamina to do as much with the house or for her husband, and she was beginning feel very limited as to what she could do as a teacher because of the fatigue and anxiety caused by lack of proper rest. Before long, Janice slipped into depression and had all but given up hope about getting better.

When she came to me, I introduced her to some natural nutrients that might be of some benefit to her. She began to take 800 I.U. of vitamin E, 1,000 mg of vitamin C, and 25,000 I.U. of beta carotene on a daily basis, along with 50 mg of coenzyme Q10 and a combination of magnesium and malic acid. On the advice of a nutritionist, she changed her eating patterns drastically and began to exercise again—walking fifteen to twenty minutes per day. Over a period of four to six weeks, she progressed to the point where she was walking from forty-five minutes to one hour each day. And after about six weeks on the program, she began to realize that she was sleeping better, the pain was beginning to subside, and she was gradually moving back toward her normal activities.

After approximately six months on my program, Janice was about 90 percent back to normal, excited about life, and making continuous progress toward returning to health and vitality. And I am happy to report that dozens upon dozens of people that I have put on the program presented in this book have made progress similar to Janice's.

body deal with stress better. Remember that exercising regularly will not only reduce stress levels, but will also increase the potential for the fibromyalgia victim to move into deep sleep while resting.

• *Balance rest and relaxation with exercise and activity.* Be sure to get adequate amounts of sleep—work at sleeping peacefully by going through your relaxation exercises while visualizing your goals. Remember that rest and relaxation will help to reduce muscle tension, which will help in reducing pain. It is also important to avoid prescription tranquilizers and sleeping medications. While these may help you get to sleep, they will suppress deep sleep and often make fibromyalgia symptoms worse the next day. Alcohol or narcotic pain medications taken in the evenings have the same effect and should also be avoided.

- *Practice good stress management techniques.* Don't overextend yourself; always plan ahead for difficult tasks; and remember to ask for help whenever needed. Limit your responsibilities and activities to manageable levels. To learn how to better manage stress, consider seeing a specialist or doing research on the internet and at the library.

- *Be especially moderate with caffeine* and alcoholic beverages. Do not use drugs unless they are prescribed by your doctor. Smoking can also increase cortisol levels in the body.

- *Above all, focus on the positive.* As discussed in the previous chapter, positive thinking can do more for an ill person than many medications. There are many people who have experienced drastic change in their physical condition simply by choosing to perceive things differently. If you change your attitude, your expectations and your vision of yourself, you can change your condition and your health.

6

The Nutrition Factor

"Let your food be your medicine, let your medicine be your food." – HIPPOCRATES

In the previous chapter, I talked about the value of nutrition in the treatment of fibromyalgia. The foods that we eat either strengthen or weaken the immune system making us more or less vulnerable to the symptoms of disease such as fibromyalgia. In fact, research shows that many diseases—diabetes, heart disease, certain cancers—are linked to poor nutrition. Following the nutritional guidelines in this chapter will enhance your immune system and greatly lower your chances for fibromyalgia and other diseases. I will discuss foods that may help reverse fibromyalgia, along with the essentials of a good nutrition program, including supplements such as vitamins, minerals and antioxidants.

Balance and Variety: The Keys in Nutrition

Your body needs a variety of nutrients in order to function at peak performance, including fats, carbohydrates, protein, fiber, vitamins, minerals and phytochemicals. In fact, the body needs ninety nutrients daily, including sixty minerals, sixteen vitamins, twelve essential amino acids and three essential fatty acids. When treating fibromyalgia or any other chronic condition, it is essential to eat a variety of food amounts and combinations. If you continuously eats the same foods over and over, you may miss out on many of the important building blocks in a healthful regimen.

The lower quality of the modern diet enhances the weakening of our immune systems and increases the potential for chronic conditions such as fibromyalgia. In the past, more plants were organically grown, and soils were much richer in a wider range of essential minerals. In today's commercial agriculture, healthy plants are artificially created by the use of herbicides, fungicides, fertilizers and pesticides. When chemicals are sprayed on plants, essential soil microbes that help plants absorb minerals into their root systems are killed. It is most difficult to absorb adequate levels of the essential nutrients when they are simply not available in the soil. Therefore, we should seek out more foods that are grown organically and possess more of the vitamins and minerals without all the added chemicals (Weintraub, 1997). It may also be useful to fill in any remaining gaps by taking supplements.

If you are still not convinced about the need for supplements, consider data from the USDA which found that approximately half of the U.S. population regularly consumes a diet deficient in basic RDA nutrients. In other words, Americans are typically not consuming the minimum RDA recommendations in one or more minerals each day. On top of that, the RDAs are only meant to prevent malnutrition; they do not give dosage amounts for optimal daily nutrition.

Later in this chapter, I will outline two nutrient programs for fibromyalgia sufferers that will help rebuild and maintain the immune system. I will also describe in further detail what I consider "miracle nutrients," but first, let's take a closer look at which dietary habits offer the most health benefits.

Eating to Combat Fibromyalgia

Even though it is difficult to get the nourishment we need from diet alone, I believe that relying solely on nutritional supplements is the wrong approach. The best health plans combine the benefits of supplements with those of good eating habits. The healthiest eating pattern involves eating the right foods, but also eating smaller, more frequent meals, four to six times daily, including enjoying healthy snacks for energy and nutrition. Healthy eaters never skip breakfast. Most unhealthy and/or overweight people develop the habit of skipping breakfast. Always eat breakfast, lunch and dinner with a couple of healthy snacks in between. The following suggestions will help you adopt healthier eating habits:

- *Eat every few hours* (six times a day) to maintain energy, to avoid getting too hungry and to keep metabolism at its maximum.

- *Include snacks in your daily routine.* Nutritious snacks should be stashed both at work and at home (i.e., raw fruits and vegetables, vegetable and fruit juices, dried fruit, whole grain crackers, bagels, unsalted nuts, pretzels and popcorn without butter). If you are concerned that late morning and late afternoon snacks will ruin your appetite for the good meal, reduce your portion size—choose a piece of fruit, whole grain bread sticks or crackers, or nibble on raw vegetables. Keeping both your meals and snacks small will prevent overeating.

- *Work toward eliminating sugared cereals,* soft drinks, candy, cookies, food additives and preservatives. Doing so will allow you to quickly enhance the reversal of fibromyalgia symptoms, especially pain and lack of deep sleep.

- *Remember that everyone should eat a wide variety* of foods that contain the ninety essential nutrients I mentioned earlier.

Most people will benefit from eating more fresh fruits and vegetables, seeds, nuts, cereals and whole grains. These foods provide the necessary fiber and fluid, higher quality fats, complex carbohydrates, necessary protein and the vitamins and minerals necessary for optimal health and for combating fibromyalgia symptoms.

- *Complex carbohydrates are important* and should make up approximately 60–70 percent of your calories. Carbohydrates are, no doubt, one of the most important foods because they provide most of the fuel for the moving body and the working, healing muscles. Carbs have gotten negative attention lately, but eliminating them is not the answer. Simply choose complex carbohydrates over simple ones whenever possible. Energy is one of the primary problems with the fibromyalgia patient, and complex carbohydrates taken on a daily basis will increase and maintain a high energy level.

- *Don't forget the fat.* Fat should make up approximately 20 percent of your calories. Although fat has been named as the culprit in heart disease and obesity, certain types of fat are a necessary component in a healthful nutrition regimen. It is essential here to read your labels and get most of your fat from healthy sources, such as polyunsaturates and monounsaturates like canola, olive, safflower, peanut and corn oils.

- *Protein is also essential for balance,* and it should make up 10–15 percent of your calories. Include protein from beans, legumes, nuts, other vegetables along with chicken, turkey, tuna and fish. Focus particularly on sources of vegetable protein, which are often ignored in the typical American diet. A very good suggestion would be to have a green salad and a portion of some type of beans every day. Utilize these sources of protein rather than red meats, which may be detrimental to the fibromyalgia victim.

- *Completely eliminate junk/fast foods.* Also, avoid caffeine, sugar and any unnecessary drugs. These highly processed items are usually filled with empty calories and potentially hazardous additives and preservatives.

- *By all means use purified water,* ideally eight to ten eight-ounce glasses per day. A water purification system is highly desirable to provide the pure water for cooking and drinking. You will need to drink additional water if you exercise or spend time outdoors when it is hot.

- *Lose the additives.* It is essential to remove as many artificial food additives and chemicals as possible from your nutritional program by eating more whole foods and using a detox program, discussed in Chapters 6 and 7.

- *Avoid refined and processed foods as much as possible,* especially foods that are canned or boxed as they always have more additives. Fresh foods always have fewer additives (and sometimes none at all).

Maintaining a Healthy Weight

You may have noticed one underlying premise to the above tips: Habits that contribute to obesity may also worsen fibromyalgia symptoms. In fact, being overweight is directly related to at least sixty-seven other diseases, including high blood pressure, heart disease, diabetes, secondary osteoarthritis, fibromyalgia, stress and depression. By employing a good weight maintenance program, you may greatly improve the symptoms of fibromyalgia. Remember a healthy weight is one of the major components of your health and wellness program during the healing and recovery process.

One mistake individuals often make when trying to lose weight is trying fad diets. Following highly restrictive diets or crash diets that are based on a limited number of foods are not physiologically healthy and do not work in the long run. They are based on short-term (unhealthy) eating habits, not long-term success. On many of these diets, you will almost always lose weight initially—sometimes a great deal of weight in the first week or two—and feel that you are beginning a program on which you are highly successful. However, research studies show that people who go on stringent or highly restrictive diets usually gain their lost weight back, over and over again. These people normally become heavier over time and have a higher mortality rate than those who remain at a constant weight on a healthy weight maintenance program. This is why it is very important to make a *lifelong lifestyle change*, where you permanently adhere to healthy lifestyle prescription on a daily basis. This can really make the difference for health and longevity.

The key is to choose an easy, flexible, sensible nutrition plan that does not call for special shopping or tedious calorie counting. The following are a few guidelines to assist you along the way on your lifetime weight management program. The individuals who have lost weight successfully and kept it off have generally utilized these tips:

- *Make a commitment to change.* As I mentioned earlier, without a firm commitment, chances for change are not very likely. Vow to improve your health, lose weight and reduce the symptoms of your fibromyalgia. If this is the goal of your physician or a family member, but not your own, then it's not likely that you'll be successful. Dietary changes are particularly difficult to follow through on if you do it half-heartedly.

- *Plan ahead and be organized.* Do not eat sporadically and/or automatically. Also, do not prepare or serve more than can be eaten. Planning ahead can help prevent impulse eating—where most of our calories are consumed. Those who are successful with their programs prepare in advance for well-balanced meals at home and for upcoming events, even taking their own food to a function if necessary. Always arrange a schedule so that you have time for your exercise sessions and meals. These are two of the most important events of the day. Once again, never skip meals—especially breakfast.

- *Set challenging but realistic goals.* Goal-oriented people are usually successful with their efforts because they set attainable goals for themselves. Do not try to lose too much weight in too short a period of time, and do not set a weight loss goal that is unrealistic for your height and body type. A healthy weight loss rate is no more than two pounds per week. Setting unrealistic weight loss goals is not only unhealthy, it will also further discourage you if you fail.

- *Prepare wisely.* Prepare healthy meals by boiling, baking and steaming instead of frying. It is very important to include at least 20 percent fat in your meals, but saturated fats and fats from frying are not ideal sources.

- *Keep busy and productive.* Do not use eating to occupy leisure time, and be sure that you're exercising regularly. Keeping your body moving boosts your metabolic rate allowing you to burn calories all day, even hours after your exercise session—and even when you are resting. Regular exercise will increase your lean body tissue and decrease your body fat tissue, and increased muscle mass means increased calorie needs, which also boosts your metabolism.

- *Beware of social binges.* Eat wisely at functions and avoid refrigerator raids. Many foods at social functions contain "hidden" calories, especially soft drinks and alcohol. If you drink alcohol at all, and especially at social functions, be sure that it's used in great moderation. This is very important to your weight maintenance program and most vital to your healing process from your fibromyalgia.

- *Monitor your progress and reward your accomplishments.* Keep track of percent body fat (also called body-mass index or BMI) and your weight loss in inches and pounds about once a week. Do not be concerned with weighing and measuring on a daily basis. Remember that people who are successful at losing and maintaining their weight and improving their health do not follow stringent or crash diets; nor do they burden themselves with calorie counting. Focus on total health and getting well. Do not be so concerned with numbers on the scale or how much farther you can walk each day. Simply allow those things to happen naturally as you are getting healthier, feeling better and getting well.

- *Practice effective stress management techniques.* Learn deep breathing and muscle relaxation exercises. If you need to, go to a professional to learn how. Be organized and efficient with time, as this is one major stress reliever. Remember to get seven to eight hours of sleep every night, always retiring at the same time to establish a pattern of effective and efficient sleep. Include a minimum of two (and possibly three) fifteen-minute relaxation sessions on a daily basis. This will add tremendously to your health and vitality, and to your recovery.

- *Develop a positive success attitude.* Concentrate on succeeding and not negative past habit patterns or failures. Avoid negative environments and negative people who will not be supportive. Focus on why you have developed poor eating habits and what those poor habits were, times of day you were eating, what you were eating and how you were preparing. Finally, make a conscious effort to change those behaviors.

Now that I have discussed the importance of maintaining a healthy weight, let's look at the nuts and bolts of good nutrition for reversing fibromyalgia.

Nutrition Protocol for Fibromyalgics

Just how critical are nutrition and natural supplements to the health and wellness process? Well, consider for a moment how the body regenerates. Did you know that every six to eight months your total body (bones, organs, skin, cells) has been made anew, recreated? As you are reading this, old cells are degenerating and dying, as new cells are being regenerated to replace those. And what do you suppose helps the body create new healthy cells? Think about it. No matter what the autoimmune problem, disease, or systemic condition, by having the knowledge and doing the right things consistently you can get better, have more energy, get rid of pain, and return to health and vitality by regenerating or recreating new cells.

For instance, fibromyalgia sufferers worldwide are told that they cannot get well—that is simply not true. Let's take the problem of muscle pain as an example. If we are recreating new muscle fiber every six to eight months, then who is to say that we can't rid ourselves of our current faulty muscle fiber and change our eating habits, exercise habits and other lifestyle patterns, so we can regenerate strong, healthy, pain-free muscle fiber?

The answer is emphatically that *we absolutely can.* You have already read the results from some of those I have had the privilege of working with from around the world. In addition to the examples in the book, there are dozens upon dozens who have gotten (or are currently getting) their lives and health back on track.

And the wonderful news is, it doesn't have to be complicated. One of my joys as a teacher is to share with you the proper education you need to reverse fibromyalgia, simply and easily. If you follow every component of my program, you will succeed.

My recommended nutrition protocol is designed for success. The grocery shopping and food preparation is simple because there are no obscure food items or complicated menus. Healthy eating does not have to involve stringent calorie counting or restrictive dieting. In fact, you may have already noticed that my advice is really just a collection of basic concepts for good nutrition. This chapter is really meant to remind you about a lot of concepts you probably already know but may have forgotten to incorporate into your life.

My program helps to resolve trauma, pain and inflammation by lowering the impact of damaging toxins and free radicals and by stimulating the building and healing process. The body is the engine, and nutrition is the fuel. As you change your lifestyle and become more active, you must feed the body what it needs to refurbish for health, healing and regeneration. You can see by looking at the accompanying "Fibromyalgia Power Foods" chart (see sidebar) that you can eat well and have plenty of tasty foods while becoming healthier—without the use of drugs, weight-loss powders or starvation.

This chart will help you to more easily choose the proper portions of proteins, carbohydrates and fats as you plan your meals. Simply choose a food from each column in any combination. For example, a sample meal could include grilled salmon (protein), steamed wild rice (carbohydrate) with broccoli (vegetable), green salad with sesame oil (good fat) and vinegar. There are literally dozens of meals that can be designed from the Power Foods lists. (For more sample meals, see Appendix B.)

Power Foods

As you can see, the "Fibromyalgia Power Foods" chart (see sidebar) offers a variety of healthy food choices to counteract the effects of fibromyalgia and other illnesses. Power foods boost immune and other body functions and buffer us against various diseases, including cancer, heart disease, diabetes, fibromyalgia and other systemic conditions. This section discusses the benefits of some of these power foods in more detail.

Fibromyalgia Power Foods

Protein	Carbohydrates	Vegetables	Fats
10–15%*	60–70%*		15–20%*
Salmon	Pasta	Cabbage	Olive oil
Tuna	Oatmeal	Cauliflower	Canola oil
Chicken breast	Strawberries	Red peppers	Sesame oil
Shrimp	Corn	Green peppers	Fish oil
Lobster	Apples	Tomato	Flaxseed oil
Turkey breast	Sweet potato	Peas	Evening primrose oil
Crab	Baked potato	Spinach	
Haddock	Yams	Cucumber	Essential fatty acids (EFAs)
Orange roughy	Squash	Zucchini	
Lean beef	Pumpkin	Celery	Sunflower seeds
Sirloin steak	Barley	Onion	
Lean ham	Melon	Kale	
Butter beans	Banana	Carrots	
Egg whites	Mango	Green beans	
Low-fat cottage cheese	Brown rice	Asparagus	
	Wild rice	Broccoli	
	Whole-wheat bread	Brussels sprouts	

Pick proteins and carbohydrates from the columns above for each meal.
Choose a serving of vegetables for at least two meals a day.
* Represents daily percentage needed

Power Proteins

Beans

We get much of our fiber from beans, which helps to regulate blood sugar levels, staves off hunger and also reduces a diabetic's need for insulin. Beans are also thought to lower blood pressure. Beans are an excellent source of plant protein.

Egg Whites/Egg Substitutes

Athletes have long utilized egg whites as a source of protein. Egg substitutes such as eggbeaters are also an excellent choice. Just be certain that eggs are cooked properly to protect against salmonella.

Fish/Seafood

Seafood is an excellent protein source. Shellfish like shrimp, crab and lobster are high in protein and low in fat, and fish such as perch, snapper, grouper, halibut, salmon, cod, tuna and swordfish are excellent choices, especially if grilled or baked. Fresh or canned white chunk tuna (packed in water) is also an excellent protein choice.

Lentils

In addition to vegetable protein, lentils provide a bonanza of nutrients, especially B-complex vitamins. One particular study suggests that they protect against heart attacks because they are very high in fiber, protein and minerals such as iron and immune-boosting copper, manganese and zinc.

Poultry

The breasts of chicken and turkey are good choices for low-fat, high-protein foods, if grilled or baked with the skin removed. You can also roast or sauté them for tasty meals. Be careful of ground turkey or chicken because very often butchers will include dark meat, skin and possibly some ingredients you don't really want to know about. Because of preservatives and additives, packaged meats are also less desirable. For a less traditional poultry choice, consider ostrich, which is low in fat, calories and cholesterol and tastes like beef.

Red Meat

Although daily beef consumption for fibromyalgia patients is discouraged, very lean beef is a super source of zinc, an immune system strengthener, and also contains niacin, which may help prevent cancerous conditions. Lean beef will also protect against cell damage that can lead to cancer and helps to fend off infections. So, red meat may be eaten in moderation if certain guidelines are followed. Lean meat is high in protein and only about 6 to 8 percent fat. Some of the better choices are top sirloin, chuck, flank and top round cuts.

Coronary artery disease continues to top the charts as the leading cause of death in the United States, but surprisingly, the fat and cholesterol in lean red meat are not the major cause. In fact, skinned chicken breast contains 72 mg of fat, fish such as flounder contains 58 mg, while top round steak contains 70 mg. The truth is that the major contributors to heart disease are lack of exercise (aerobic) and the overconsumption of saturated fat.

Other sources of red meat include venison (deer) and buffalo.

Skim Milk

Research studies show that postmenopausal women who take 150 mg of calcium (in supplement form) daily reduce their bone loss. Researchers are now convinced that extra calcium can absolutely strengthen bones and prevent fractures in older adults. Skim milk appears to be one of the best sources of bone-building calcium and riboflavin. (Riboflavin is a B vitamin that helps maintain energy.)

Soy

Soy is an invaluable power food and a complete vegetable protein. Research studies have shown that populations with high soy intake have lowered rates of heart disease, osteoporosis and breast cancer.

Yogurt

Yogurt has been proven in research studies to prevent allergies and colds. Researchers at the University of California at Davis found that people who ate an eight-ounce carton of yogurt with live cultures (specifically *Lactobacillus*, *Bulgaricus* and *Streptococcus thermophilous*) daily had 25 percent fewer colds and almost ten times fewer allergy symptoms than those eating the same amount of yogurt with "killed" cultures. Yogurt is a great source of calcium as well. Other research studies have also borne out that yogurt lowers cholesterol. Look for live cultures listed on the containers.

Power Carbohydrates

Fruit

Fruits are especially rich in nutrients, and the good news is that the sugar in fruits (fructose) is in its natural form. Most fruits also have a very low glycemic index score. Fruits are carbohydrates that can be easily combined with a portion of protein for a meal. They also have many beneficial nutrients.

Apricots. Apricots are loaded with antioxidants, beta carotene and vitamin C. Researchers have recently established that vitamin C can help prevent cataracts along with reducing the risk of cancers of the mouth, throat, stomach and pancreas. Apricots are also packed with fiber and when combined with a low-fat diet, they can lessen the risk of colon polyps.

Bananas. Bananas may help to lower blood pressure. They are high in vitamin B6 and rich in potassium. Research indicates that they are essential to building a strong immune system.

Cantaloupe. Cantaloupe is packed with vitamin C, fiber, folic acid, potassium, beta carotene and vitamin B6.

Grapes. Grapes are an excellent source of boron, a mineral that helps to prevent osteoporosis. Red grape juice also contains *resveratrol*, a phytochemical that may help prevent heart disease by inhibiting the "clumping" of blood cells.

Kiwi. Kiwi is literally packed with vitamin C and cancer-fighting fiber.

Mangos. Mangos are packed with vitamin B6, copper and anticancer antioxidants like beta carotene and vitamin C. The combination of these antioxidants have been shown in a USDA study to lower blood pressure.

Orange Juice. All citrus fruits and juices, including orange juice, contain liminoids. These are substances that research studies have shown can activate detoxifying enzymes in the body, which reduce cancer risk. Orange juice is a classic source of vitamin C, and it is recommended that smokers take twice the amount that nonsmokers require because nicotine leeches vitamin C from the body. So if you have fibromyalgia, quit smoking!

Pears. Pears provide vitamin C, potassium, boron and fiber.

Prunes. Prunes are a source of bone-saving boron and the antioxidant vitamins A and E, and they are loaded with fiber.

Strawberries. Strawberries offer more vitamin C and fiber than many other fruits. Strawberries also contain elegiac acid, which is a natural cancer-fighting chemical.

Potatoes

Almost everyone's favorite carbohydrate is the potato. Fortunately, mother nature has cooperated with us—potatoes are nature made in portion sizes. To choose a good healthy portion, just find a potato about the size of your clenched fist.

When we eat potatoes we are tempted to pour on the sour cream and butter; however, potatoes taste great just by themselves, and if you don't believe me just try it. If you choose add a little butter, then use real butter. Margarines contain trans fats that are unhealthy.

Sweet Potatoes or Yams

Sweet potatoes and yams are one of the better choices of carbohydrates and are absolutely loaded with nutrients. Most people have the misconception that sweet potatoes are higher in calories than the regular potatoes, but this is not true. The sweet taste in a sweet potato is the result of an enzyme that converts starches into sugars and, therefore, makes the potato taste very sweet, but they are a great source of fiber. In fact, sweet potatoes contain almost twice the fiber and much more beta carotene than white and red potatoes.

Baking, boiling or microwaving are some of the better ways to prepare sweet potatoes. Something to remember when you bring them home from the grocery store: do not refrigerate them or they become hard and bitter tasting. A better choice is to store them in a dry cool place where they will keep for several weeks.

Whole Grains

All whole-grain foods are very rich in vitamin B6, fiber and manganese. Whole-wheat bread for instance contains triple the fiber of white bread. Everyone needs extra B6 as we age to keep our immune systems strong.

Barley. Barley is probably one of the healthiest carbohydrate foods available. It can be hard to find in the grocery store, but you can usually pick it up at the health food store. Barley also has one of the lowest glycemic index scores on the carbohydrate list. Barley comes in pearl or flake form and can be cooked and eaten as a hot cereal. It can be a bit bland, but with some cinnamon or brown sugar, it is very tasty. Barley can also replace rice in a dinner meal.

Bran Cereal. This cereal is very high in wheat bran and is one of the best sources of cancer-fighting insoluble fiber—the kind of fiber that increases stool bulk and speed. Bran cereal provides about five grams of fiber per serving.

Brown Rice. The big difference between brown rice and white rice is the way they are processed. Processed white rice changes the way the body uses its carbohydrates. Carbohydrates are the main source of fuel for our bodies, and brown rice burns much slower than white rice. In other words, brown rice will give you more energy for a longer period of time than white rice.

A portion of a quality protein and a portion of steamed brown rice with a vegetable make a great meal. The high-fiber bran in brown rice can help lower cholesterol. Brown rice is very high in vitamin B6 and magnesium. The benefits of these two nutrients for fibromyalgia patients cannot be emphasized enough. Brown rice also provides thiamine (vital for nerve function), niacin, copper and zinc. Research studies indicate that vitamin E from brown rice tends to strengthen the immune system and will reduce the risk of heart disease and cataracts.

Pasta. Surprise! Pasta is a low glycemic index food even though it is not a whole grain. The durum wheat from semolina flour that's used to make most dried pastas is not broken down as quickly as other flours. Pastas such as linguini, spaghetti and macaroni are good sources of carbohydrates. The key to making pasta work for you is to recognize the difference between a huge helping and a portion. One serving of pasta is approximately half a cup. Also, when you do eat pasta, choose small portions of sauces, and be careful of butter, alfredo sauce and cheese if you are watching calories. In fact, you could simply squeeze lemon over your pasta, as I like to do on occasion, to keep it simple yet tasty.

Oatmeal. Oats lower LDL (bad) cholesterol. Research studies have found that if individuals eat three grams of soluble fiber a day, which is about the amount found in three packets of instant oatmeal, one can lower LDL cholesterol by 6 percent within six weeks.

Oatmeal is obviously an old favorite for many. Be cautious in your selection, however, as there are several high-sugar, instant oatmeals that should be avoided. Instead, choose all-natural, rolled oats that are not processed and do not contain sugar.

Rolled oats are a low glycemic index food, meaning that they are converted to blood sugar much slower than most processed foods. This helps control blood sugar levels and makes them an excellent choice for efficient weight loss and/or maintenance and overall health. Use some cinnamon or brown sugar for taste. Oatmeal is also a great source of fiber and may help prevent heart disease.

Wheat Germ. Wheat germ is an excellent source of many nutrients. Just one-fourth cup will provide as much as five grams of fiber as well as almost all of the daily requirements of magnesium, zinc, iron and B-complex vitamins. Wheat germ is incredibly rich in manganese, and it is also one of the best sources of chromium and vitamin E.

Whole-wheat Bread. Many people attempt to eliminate breads altogether, and in my opinion, that is not absolutely necessary. In fact, one of my favorite meals is a turkey or grilled chicken sandwich. The key here is to choose unprocessed, whole-grain bread for your sandwich. Just remember to be moderate with breads and wise in your selection.

Power Fats

One major error made by most dieters is thinking that all fats are bad and trying to eliminate all fats from their meals. The truth is that there are good fats and there are bad fats, with saturated fats and trans fats being the worst. In fact, unsaturated fats in moderate amounts can actually be good for you.

Let's take fish, for example. Fish is an extremely healthy food because it contains essential fatty acids, often referred to as EFAs, that can assist your body in burning fat more efficiently and protect you from many diseases.

How do you know which fats are good? A good rule to follow for knowing which fats are okay is knowing if the fat becomes solid at room temperature, like butter, margarine or shortening. If so, the fat is bad news.

A short list of good fats would include olive oil, canola oil, omega-3 fish oil, sesame oil, flaxseed oil and evening primrose oil. You can take around a tablespoon a day and provide your body with all the essential fatty acids it needs. For instance, you can take a tablespoon of olive oil and mix it together with a little vinegar for a salad dressing, or you can eat a portion of fish about three times a week to get all the essential fatty acids you need to be healthy.

Fish Oil

The essential fatty acids in fish oils have been found to lower triglycerides (blood fats and sugars). High levels of triglycerides are thought to be more harmful to women than men. It is recommended that fish should be eaten three to four times a week.

Lake trout, salmon, sardines, anchovies, herring and blue fish are those that have the most essential fatty acids.

Nuts

Nuts are heart helpers. For example, adults on a low-fat diet who ate two ounces of walnuts, five or more times a week, lowered their cholesterol levels by 12 percent.

Olive Oil

Olive oil is a key component of the healthy Mediterranean diet. Olive oil is the oil richest in monounsaturated fats, which have been shown to lower cholesterol.

Sunflower Seeds

Sunflower seeds are high in vitamin E, an antioxidant that fights heart disease, cancer and cataracts. Sunflower seeds are also very similar to nuts in polyunsaturated fat content.

Power Vegetables

Vegetables are not only high in fiber, they are also low in calories and are power packed with nutrients and antioxidants, which have proven through research to help prevent most systemic conditions as well as cancer. One study found a link between vegetable consumption and rheumatoid arthritis risk, and another found that a vegan diet may reduce incidence of joint pain. Be careful not to overload your veggies with cheese, butter or deep frying. Ideally, you would buy your veggies fresh or frozen and eat as many of them as possible lightly steamed or raw to preserve beneficial nutrients and enzymes. Remember that raw fruits and veggies are some of the best cleansers or detoxifiers.

These are healthy, high-nutrient foods that should be included in at least two of your daily meals: cauliflower, cabbage, green and red bell peppers, spinach, cucumber, peas, tomatoes, zucchini, kale, carrots, onions, celery, Brussels sprouts, asparagus, broccoli, mushrooms and green beans.

Broccoli

Broccoli contains potassium and chromium, which stabilize blood sugar. Broccoli is also filled with cancer-fighting fiber, vitamin C, beta carotene, bone-building calcium, folic acid, boron and sulforaphane, which detoxifies harmful enzymes in the body.

Cabbage

Substances called "indols" in cabbage are anticancer agents.

Carrots

Scientific studies suggest that one carrot a day may reduce lung cancer risk in ex-smokers. Carrots are also loaded with beta carotene.

Garlic

Garlic helps to protect against heart disease and stroke. It might also lower blood pressure, and it acts as a natural antibiotic. Research studies suggest that garlic has multiple benefits, including the fact that it appears to defuse carcinogenic chemicals (e.g. those from cigarettes).

Kale

Kale is packed with fiber, calcium, manganese, vitamin B6, copper and potassium. Kale also reduces the harmful effects of the LDL cholesterol.

Pumpkin

Pumpkin is particularly high in beta carotene and fiber.

Red Bell Peppers

Red bell peppers are a better anticancer choice than green peppers because they contain added carotenes. Red bell peppers also supply powerful antioxidant properties and help fight cancer by inhibiting the formation of carcinogenic nitrosamines (formed when you ingest foods containing nitrates such as bacon, sausage and cured beef).

Spinach

Spinach provides a powerhouse of antioxidants and is very rich is folic acid.

Tomatoes

Tomatoes contain lycopene, a chemical also found in pink grapefruit and thought to help prevent some cancers, including prostate cancer. Tomatoes are also an excellent source of vitamins A and C, as well as fiber and potassium.

Other Power Foods

Ginger

Ginger is a spice, and like many other spices including rosemary, pepper, oregano and thyme, it is a powerful antioxidant.

Tea

Worldwide studies have suggested that the chemicals in tea tend to prevent cancer and lower blood cholesterol.

More Meal Planning Advice

Don't get caught up with the misconception that healthy high-nutrient meals have to be tasteless, bland and boring—that is absolutely not the case. If you follow my program, meals can be tasty, fun and energizing. Most of the meals are simple to prepare, and more importantly, they will provide your body with the quality nutrition that you need to regenerate cells that are going to bring you back to total health.

You may be of the opinion that eating six times a day can be difficult, cumbersome and even expensive. But when you really think about it, if you plan well, then it is relatively easy to do. In fact, in Appendix B I have included some meal planning ideas and charts to help you organize. Below are some additional suggestions that take the guessing and difficulty out of following a healthy nutritional program.

Snack Options

At the beginning of this chapter, I mentioned a few snack ideas to help you meet the six-meal requirement. Although processed or packaged snack items may seem easier than healthier options, there are countless nutritious snacks that are just as simple. Fresh veggies or fruit make a great snack, as does yogurt with granola or low-fat cottage cheese with fruit. Unsalted nuts are another great option, and many grocery stores offer healthy trail mixes that also make great snacks. A small tuna fish sandwich on whole-wheat bread is another option, or if you want something a little lighter, try a fresh-made fruit or veggie juice—or a fruit smoothie.

Despite these options, I know that sometimes schedules are too hectic for even the simplest whole-food snacks, especially when you can't plan in advance. On busy days, you may want to try a nutritional drink or bar for one or two of your meals. Slimfast and Vita-trim are two brands that offer both bars and drinks in a variety of flavors. There are also a number of soy drinks now on the market that are tasty and more nutritious. There are also powder shakes available that you can use to make smoothies or other health drinks by adding fruit, fruit juice, soy powder, wheat germ or other health additives.

These options give you an alternative to traditional snack foods and may increase your chance for success on a day-to-day basis. Especially for those of you who are not accustomed to eating small and frequent high-nutrient meals day-in and day-out. They are also great meals after a strenuous workout.

Be a Grocery Shopping Planner

The old saying is, "when you fail to plan then you plan to fail." Always make a list and plan ahead before going to the grocery store to assure that your pantry and refrigerator are stocked with choice foods. Use the power foods lists, plan ahead, and make your grocery list so that you will consistently eat better. Many times we think that packaged foods are easier because we do not take the time to plan our meals and snacks beforehand. Even planning one day in advance can make a huge difference. Meal planning will enable you to have greater success in sticking with a healthy diet and reversing fibromyalgia.

The "Bonus Day" Concept

The purpose of eating six meals a day and following the outlined program is to consistently keep your metabolism revved up throughout the day so that your body becomes more efficient in burning calories, burning fat, and continuously moving you toward your goal of restored health. So what do we mean by a bonus day? Six days a week I want you to follow the guidelines that I have given you here, and then once a week, you can have a bonus day, meaning that on the seventh day, you can eat anything and everything that you wish.

Some of the things I have learned over the many years of working with people and doing research is that if there are too many rigid guidelines, then they are set up to fail. Most people need some leeway that allows them to make some decisions for themselves. Most individuals are very amenable to structure and framework as long as there is some freedom left within that structure. At some point after the 21-day detox period I discuss in the next chapter, as your body rids itself of junk food, sweets, toxins and other unhealthy foods, you will come to the realization that you don't need to overeat these foods nor will you crave them.

There are biological and physiological reasons for allowing the bonus day. For instance the ingrained DNA structure that has been there for centuries is impacted if you loosen-up and eat more at least once a week. The bonus day assists you in convincing your body that it is not being starved. The bonus day will also serve an important purpose in reminding you of what it feels like to overeat, stuff yourself, to become sluggish, have an energy drain and indigestion—all the things created by overeating and eating improperly.

The Day-Planning Log

I am also providing you with a day-planning log (see Appendix B) so you can plan all six meals each day ahead of time. On the left side of your chart, you have a place to plan your meals and what you would like to attempt to do. Then, on the right side your chart is a place to record what you actually did. When you can see these results, it will give you some sense of satisfaction that you are staying on track and accomplishing your goals, not to mention the fact that you are assuring yourself that you have the proper amount and proportions of carbohydrates, protein, healthy fats and veggies.

Tracking what you eat, when you eat, the supplements you take, etc., can be beneficial in taking full advantage of your nutritional plan. To help you do this, I have provided a notes/diary section on the log sheet where you can note your eating habits, supplement plan, exercise regimen and other elements of your strategy on a daily basis. This section can be used to document pain intensity, stress levels and management, medications, questions for your physician and any other notes that will help you on your road to recovery.

Correct the Carbohydrate Misconception

My research and experience over the past twenty-five years indicate to me that the *Atkins Protein Diet* and the *Zone Diet* are way off base when they portray carbohydrates as the culprit in our diets, and many nutrition experts agree. For healthy weight loss and for overall health, it is advisable to eat more, not fewer carbohydrates. The key is to be careful about your choice of carbohydrates. Be careful about refined carbs and sugars as opposed to the more nutritious complex carbohydrates like whole grains. The better and more scientific programs divide carbohydrates into good and bad categories, depending on the effect they have on your body. The determining factor is the rapidity with which carbohydrates are broken down into glucose, or ready-to-use blood sugar as our primary fuel source. The bottom line is that a healthy, active body needs a larger percentage of carbohydrates. (The exception is the diabetic, who is forced to reduce carbs to a degree.)

To determine the speed of carbohydrate breakdown, nutrition scientists use a rating scale called the "glycemic index" (GI). How rapid carbohydrates are changed to glucose depends on many factors, and one of those key factors is how much fiber is in the food. The more fiber in a particular food, the slower it takes to break down, and thus, the healthier the food is for the body. Some of the better foods are whole grains, fruits, vegetables, beans and legumes. These are generally low GI foods, meaning they are broken down very slowly and release a steady supply of glucose into the blood. This simply means that complex carbohydrates with more fiber cleanse our systems more efficiently, and they give us enough staying power to curb hunger until its time for the next meal. Some of the more simple, refined carbs such as pretzels, rice cakes, bagels and white bread have very high GI scores, meaning they are converted to glucose very quickly and trigger a sharp rise in the flow of insulin, the hormone that moves glucose from the blood stream to the cells for energy.

Insulin levels are the key, according to the experts. Continually high insulin levels that are created by the highly refined foods lead to weight gain and blood sugar irregularities. If your insulin levels are high, you will have trouble burning fat for energy and will have trouble losing weight. So then, the key to health, healthy weight loss and weight maintenance, is to

Pick the Right Carbs

The glycemic index (GI) ranks foods on a scale of 0 to 100, depending on how fast they're digested and converted to glucose. Below are the scores for some popular carbohydrate foods. Emphasize low-scoring GI foods in your diet, but remember, you can also have some high GI foods if you eat them in moderation.

Food	GI Score	Food	GI Score	Food	GI Score
Barley	25	Oatmeal, rolled oats	49	Potatoes, new	62
Grapefruit	25	Bread, 100% stone		Raisins	64
Kidney beans	27	ground whole wheat	53	Cantaloupe	65
Lentils	30	Buckwheat	54	Couscous	65
Fettuccine	32	Sweet potato	54	Bread, whole wheat	69
Apple	38	Corn	55	Bread, white	70
Pear	38	Popcorn	55	Bagel	72
Peach	42	Rice, brown	55	Graham crackers	74
Orange	44	Apricot	57	Rice cakes	82
Grapes, green	46	Bread, whole-wheat		Pretzels	83
Linguine	46	pita	57	Cornflakes	84
Bulgur		Rice, basmati	58	Potatoes, baked	85
(cracked wheat)	48			Rice, instant white	87

choose complex carbs with more fiber, the power proteins, power fats, fruits and veggies (as outlined in my nutrition protocol). To assist you with choosing good carbohydrates with low GI scores, use the chart in the accompanying sidebar "Pick the Right Carbs." For more information, refer to the book, *The Glucose Revolution*.

What's Wrong with Sugar?

Empty sugar calories provided from sucrose usually crowd out nutritious foods, and they do not provide vitamins, minerals or fiber. Manufacturers advertise that their sugar products will provide quick energy, but the quick energy is very short-lived because about twenty minutes after consumption, an individual will feel cranky, tired, sluggish and sometimes even mildly depressed because of blood sugar fluctuations. If you eat snacks between meals that frequently include candy and sugared sodas, you are paving the way for poor health and opening the door for systemic conditions such as fibromyalgia.

Is Sugar Addictive?

The answer to this question is a certain "yes." Sugar acts like a drug when eaten in large amounts or if consumed daily. Sugar is one of the most damaging and destructive items in our daily diets. It is one of the primary culprits in destroying the ability of the immune system to retain its strength. Some suggested sweeteners that are healthier for those who really desire or need sweeteners are pure maple syrup, rice syrup, molasses, sucanat, honey, date sugar or stevia (Weintraub, 1996).

Comparing the Various Types of Sugars

Sugar in any form is very quickly absorbed into the blood stream and provides quick energy for the body. However, white

Summary of the Body Advantage Nutrition Principles

- Eat six mini-meals a day.
- Boil, broil, bake and steam. (Fry sparingly.)
- Plan your shopping and meals.
- Take supplements to ensure that you are getting the necessary nutrients for health and healing.
- Balance protein, carbohydrates and fats daily.
- Fruits and vegetables should be a part of at least two meals daily.
- Drink twelve cups of purified water daily.
- A portion of protein and carbohydrates should be chosen with each meal.
- A portion is the size of the palm of your hand.
- Record what you eat using the daily log in Appendix B.
- Take in one tablespoon of unsaturated oil daily or three portions of fresh salmon weekly.
- You have one bonus day per week to eat whatever you want. (Another reason why it is important to record what you eat and when.)

sugar, whether it be from sugar cane, sugar beets or corn, is completely refined, has no nutritional value and provides only empty calories. All the sugars are treated the same by the body, converting them all to glucose, whether they are sucrose, fructose or dextrose. Once converted to glucose, sugars are circulated through the bloodstream as an energy source and stored in the liver and the muscles as fat. Just a note to remember here is that most fruit juices are as sweet as candy—even the unsweetened juices. They are very high in natural sugars and very often have the same harmful effects as pure sugar candy or other sweets.

The Nutrient Rebuilding Program

If you remember, earlier in the chapter I talked about the need for nutritional supplementation. Making the dietary changes I recommend is only one part of nutritional healing. For complete success, you must at least consider taking a multi-nutrient supplement or a series of individual supplements. The following table of essential nutrients and recommended amounts will reduce stress and trauma, and resolve pain and inflammation, while lowering the impact of damaging toxins and free radicals to stimulate the rebuilding and healing process.

This immune-boosting regimen has proven effective for helping to protect against systemic conditions such as colds, flu, viruses (Epstein-Barr), chlamydial diseases, cancer, aids, lupus, mononucleosis, herpes simplex (fever blisters), herpes zoster (shingles), hypothyroidism, arthritis, chronic fatigue, as well as fibromyalgia. This rebuilding program should be followed for approximately six months before moving to the maintenance program:

Essential Nutrient	Recommended Dosage
Beta Carotene	15,000–25,000 IUs
Vitamin B1 (Thiamine)	25 milligrams
Vitamin B2 (Riboflavin)	25 milligrams
Vitamin B3 (Niacin)	25 milligrams
Vitamin B6 (Pyridoxine)	20 milligrams
Vitamin B12 (Cyanocobalamin)	200 micrograms
Boron	5 milligrams
Choline	100 milligrams
Folic Acid	200 micrograms
Biotin	200 micrograms
Inositol	50 milligrams
Vitamin C (Ascorbic Acid)	1,000–3,000 milligrams
Vitamin E (d-Alpha Tocopherol)	400–800 IUs

Malic Acid	400–800 milligrams
Magnesium (Oxide)	400 milligrams
Chromium	200 micrograms
Manganese (Amino Acid Chelate)	4 milligrams
Selenium	100 micrograms
Zinc	50 milligrams
Calcium	200 milligrams
Potassium	100 milligrams
Pycnogenol (Grape Seed Extract)	50 milligrams
Glucosamine Hydrochloride	1,500 milligrams
Bovine Cartilage (Chondroitin Sulfates)	400 milligrams
Transfer Factor (Concentrated transfer factors from bovine colostrum)	300 milligrams
Citrus Bioflavonoids	250–1,000 milligrams
Coenzyme Q10	50 milligrams

The Nutrient Maintenance Program

You will note below that the dosages of certain nutrients are reduced since not quite as much is required in your maintenance program as in the prior rebuilding program. After about six months of using the rebuilding program, you may move to the maintenance program. If you have a fibromyalgia flare-up, you may want to move back to the rebuilding program for its duration.

Essential Nutrient	*Recommended Dosage*
Beta Carotene	15,000 IUs
Vitamin B1 (Thiamine)	25 milligrams
Vitamin B2 (Riboflavin)	25 milligrams
Vitamin B3 (Niacin)	25 milligrams
Vitamin B6 (Pyridoxine)	20 milligrams
Vitamin B12 (Cyanocobalamin)	200 micrograms
Boron	5 milligrams

Choline	50 milligrams
Folic Acid	200 micrograms
Biotin	200 micrograms
Inositol	50 milligrams
Vitamin C (Ascorbic Acid)	1,000–3,000 milligrams
Vitamin E (d-Alpha Tocopherol)	400–800 IUs
Malic Acid	400 milligrams
Magnesium (Oxide)	400 milligrams
Chromium	200 micrograms
Manganese (Amino Acid Chelate)	2 milligrams
Selenium	50 micrograms
Zinc	30 milligrams
Calcium	200 milligrams
Potassium	100 milligrams
Pycnogenol (Grape Seed Extract)	50 milligrams
Glucosamine Hydrochloride	800 milligrams
Bovine Cartilage (Chondroitin Sulfates)	200 milligrams
Transfer Factor (Concentrated transfer factors from bovine colostrum)	300 milligrams
Citrus Bioflavonoids	250–1,000 milligrams
Coenzyme Q10	50 milligrams

Miracle Nutrients

Some of the nutrients recommended in the rebuilding and maintenance programs I consider "miracle nutrients" for fibromyalgia sufferers. Below is a more detailed discussion of some of these miracle nutrients:

• *Beta carotene.* There are dozens of carotenoids, including beta carotene, the plant form of vitamin A. The better sources of carotenoids are yellow and orange fruits and vegetables such as carrots, cantaloupe, sweet potatoes, pumpkin, apricots and melons such as mango, papaya, peaches and winter squash. The dark green leafy vegetables are another

"I am resting better at night"

I began the regimen outlined in your book and I have seen some improvement. The pain in my shoulder is better, my muscles do not ache as much, and my morning stiffness is improved. I am also resting better at night. I am happy to know that there is help for me with this problem.

Elaine
Tennessee

excellent source of beta carotene. Examples are collard greens, parsley, spinach, broccoli and other leafy greens.

- *Vitamin C.* This is one of the more powerful antioxidants, and the major sources are fresh fruits such as grapefruit, strawberries, bananas, cantaloupe, papaya, kiwi, mango, raspberries, pineapple and tomatoes, as well as fresh vegetables such as cabbage, asparagus, broccoli, Brussels sprouts, collard greens, potatoes and red peppers. Vitamin C is heat sensitive and easily destroyed by refining or overprocessing, and therefore, should be steamed or microwaved for a very short period of time.

- *Vitamin E.* The better sources for this powerful antioxidant are vegetable oils, especially safflower, avocados, nuts, sunflower seeds, wheat germ, whole-grain cereals and breads, asparagus, dried prunes and broccoli.

- *Selenium.* There is much evidence to substantiate selenium as an immune booster. It works by protecting cells from the toxic effects of free radicals. Some of the better food sources of selenium are shrimp, sunflower seeds, wheat breads, tuna and salmon.

- *Zinc.* This trace mineral assists in performing many vital body functions. For instance, it helps with the absorption of vitamins in the body and helps form skin, nails and hair, as well as being an essential part of many enzymes involved in metabolism and digestion. Vitamin A must be present for zinc to be properly absorbed in the body. Some excellent sources of zinc are ginseng, chalk and the herb licorice.

- *Manganese.* A trace mineral essential for the proper functioning of the pituitary gland as well as healthy functioning of the body's other glands. It is essential in the treatment of fibromyalgia because it aids glucose utilization in the process of creating energy, and it also helps the central nervous system function normally.

- *Magnesium.* This is a very essential part of the enzyme system and is most important in the rehabilitation of fibromyalgia patients. Almost 100 percent of the fibromyalgia victims I have worked with have exhibited a magnesium deficiency. Magnesium is involved in the absorption of potassium, calcium, phosphorus, and B-complex vitamins, as well as vitamins C and E. Magnesium is also essential in ATP (energy) production.

- *Malic Acid.* Another essential ingredient in the production of energy is malic acid. It is also critical in lessening the toxic effects of aluminum. When combined with magnesium, malic acid is very effective as a cleansing and healing agent for fibromyalgia and other systemic conditions.

- *Chromium.* This trace mineral is essential for the synthesis of fatty acids and the metabolism of glucose for energy. It is also well known for its ability to increase the efficiency of insulin.

- *Boron.* This trace mineral possesses some antioxidant functions and is very important in maintaining muscular health.

Muscle/Connective Tissue and Bioflavonoids

There are literally thousands of different types of bioflavonoids. They are found in virtually all plant foods and are essential for healthy capillary walls, the metabolism of vitamin C, and for enhancing the utilization of other essential nutrients. The bioflavonoids aid fibromyalgia victims by:

- enhancing the strength of collagen in connective tissue
- strengthening muscle fiber
- buffering free radical damage
- improving the functioning ability of muscle fiber
- enhancing the energy production process
- assisting in the utilization of other nutrients by the body

Some excellent sources of bioflavonoids are fresh fruits and vegetables, seeds, nuts, legumes, whole grains, citrus fruits, onions, berries, green tea and especially fruits that contain a pit (such as plums and cherries). There are also rosehip bioflavonoids, as well as citrus bioflavonoids such as catechin, hesperidin, rutin, quercetin, milk thistle seed extract, ginkgo extracts, pycnogenol (from grape seed extract) and rice bran extract (Carper, 1995).

It assists in inhibiting cells from releasing free radicals. Cauliflower and apples are sources of boron.

- *Coenzyme Q10.* Research studies indicate that this enzyme increases a vital component of the immune system (gamma globulin). Coenzyme Q10 proves valuable in the treatment of fibromyalgia because it is a very important component for enhancing circulation and increasing energy levels.

- **Proanthocyanidins.** One of the potent sources of proanthocyanidins is pycnogenol from a grape seed extract. The pycnogenol from grape seed is a very powerful antioxidant and is fifty times stronger than vitamin E. It is also very efficient in boosting the immune system and assisting in the treatment of fibromyalgia.

- **Rice Bran Extract.** There are three polyphenols from the tocotryonols of rice bran that are 6,000 times stronger than vitamin E.

- **Glucosamine.** This supplement is the key substance that determines how many proteoglycan (water-holding) molecules are formed in cartilage. Glucosamine has been found to be very effective for the improvement of arthritic conditions. Also, in a study conducted by the Vulvodynia Project, glucosamine was used to effectively reduce sensitivity and soft-tissue pain in fibromyalgia patients.

- **Chondroitin Sulfate.** Naturally occurring substances that inhibit the enzymes that degrade cartilage while helping to attract fluid to the proteoglycan molecules.

- **Colostrum/Transfer Factors.** Transfer factor is a vital immune booster that educates immune T cells. When our immune cells become more efficient, we can more readily combat chronic systemic conditions. Transfer factor is made up of proteins from colostrum, the first milk provided by a mother cow for her new calf. The first milk contains valuable immune data meant to prepare the calf's vulnerable immune system for microbe attacks. Multiple studies have shown that colostrum transfer factors may also benefit humans.

As mentioned earlier, it is generally best to get vitamins, minerals, antioxidants and other nutrients the body needs from fresh whole foods (ideally organic foods) rather than supplements. However, proper amounts of vitamins, minerals and nutrients are very difficult to acquire from foods because of depleted soils and ingested chemicals in the form of pesticides and insecticides that interfere with proper nutrient absorption. In order to get all of the necessary nutrients in today's world, it is absolutely essential that we take supplements, especially when treating chronic conditions such as fibromyalgia.

Is nutritional supplementation really necessary for healing and health? The answer is an unequivocal "yes." A well-controlled study performed at the Shriner's Burn Trauma Center at the University of Cincinnati Medical School demonstrated conclusively that children with severe burn trauma faired far better when given extra nutritional supplementation over and above the normal "well-balanced diet" generally prescribed by practitioners. All of the children receiving the extra supplementation lived, whereas, tragically, 44 percent of children given regular treatment and a "balanced" diet alone died. The scientists in the study said, "To our knowledge this is the first controlled study to demonstrate what has been suspected and accepted for some time, that nutritional intervention improves survival."

If by virtue of your personal analysis, after having read the first half of this book, you find yourself confirming one or several of the symptoms or characteristics relating to chronic fatigue, fibromyalgia or other systemic conditions, then you are in dire need of my rebuilding/rebalancing program. And if you are susceptible to colds, flu, viruses or general tiredness, you are a prime candidate for this program.

If any of the above are the case, you are probably, like most people, eating a good amount of sugar, high fat foods and packaged processed foods with harmful additives and fillers. Your exercise habits, daily diet, normal routine and self-esteem are probably very poor. This is the typical routine that gradually, over the years, leads you to become unbalanced and to the point where you are now health wise. It's very likely that you are basically unhappy and possibly view the world as a depressing place.

Most people falling in this category will almost always exhibit one or more of the debilitating symptoms of being out of balance. This downward spiraling effect must be reversed or the immune system will eventually become weakened and overwhelmed to the point that it can no longer protect the body so that it can renew and heal itself. Those experiencing the above declining health status very often will have carried some of the unhealthy symptoms for many years, will have seen a number of doctors, and will have accumulated an extensive medical record in search of a cure for their ongoing physical and emotional problems.

Antioxidants: Vital for Your Health

Scientific researchers have established the fact that a nutritional regimen is one of the key components in safeguarding our health against chronic conditions such as fibromyalgia. One of the most widely accepted theories is that disease and debilitation of the body is caused by unstable molecules called "free radicals" that rampage through the body, attacking healthy cells and destroying healthy tissue. A free radical is a molecule that's missing an electron because of breathing polluted air, metabolizing food substances in the body and consuming unhealthy food additives, etc. These molecules that are missing electrons are not happy until they take a bite out of a healthy cell, damaging it and replacing the electron that is missing (Bucci 1994). Excessive and nonbuffered free radicals are now thought to be the basic underlying cause of all diseases, including cancer, heart disease, diabetes, arthritis, and degenerative diseases and chronic conditions such as fibromyalgia.

The good news is that the bufferers for free radicals and good health are found in the form of antioxidants. Antioxidants derive their name because they serve as antidotes to one of the free radicals most commonly found in the body—oxygen. Antioxidants buffer or stabilize the free radicals preventing them from attacking and damaging other body tissues (Nierenberg, 1996). The following discussion will reveal where we find many of these antioxidants in a healthful nutrition program in the form of vitamins, minerals, carotenoids, bioflavonoids and phytonutrients.

The more powerful antioxidant vitamins are beta carotene, vitamin C, vitamin E and vitamin B6. Some of the trace minerals that serve as powerful antioxidants are selenium, zinc, manganese, magnesium, boron and chromium. Some other powerful antioxidant and immune boosting nutrients are coenzyme Q10, proanthocyanidins or pycnogenol (from grape seeds), rice bran extract, curcumin and garlic. We will encounter antioxidants in more detail in the next chapter.

7

The Fibromyalgia Detoxification Program

"Hold yourself responsible for a higher standard than anybody else expects of you." – HENRY WARD BEECHER

"Determination is the wake-up call to the human will." – ANTHONY ROBBINS

Detoxification is the process of body and/or cell cleansing through purging of toxic buildup resultant of a combination of poor diet, ingestion of abusive substances, and stress. An abusive lifestyle, including the ingestion of excessive fat, junk foods, nicotine, caffeine, excessive alcohol and other drugs, in addition to a lack of rest and undue stress will eventually create a toxic buildup within the body that can break down the immune system.

Dr. Elrod's 21-Day Detoxification Program

I have designed the following dietary guidelines to promote body cleansing as a first step back toward health and wellness, and as a new beginning for strengthening the immune system.

Ideally a ten-day "tapering off" period of gradually reducing sugar, fat, caffeine, etc. is advised before beginning the full 21-day detoxification program. The ten-day tapering period is important in assisting the body to adjust to a new diet and to ensure success with the total program. As you can see, within a thirty-day period, the cleansing (detoxification) process will be complete, and you will be on your way back to a happy, healthy, successful lifestyle.

Things to Emphasize

These are areas that one should emphasize for a successful detoxification program:

- Increase your consumption of high-fiber foods gradually: High-fiber foods include vegetables, fresh fruits, whole grains, legumes, seeds and nuts. Be sure to include peaches, strawberries, potatoes, spinach, tomatoes, wheat and bran cereals, whole-wheat bread, rice and popcorn.
- Increase raw fruits and vegetables to 50 percent of your diet. Be sure to include cucumbers, radishes, grapefruit, apples, carrots, cantaloupe, red bell peppers and green leafy vegetables.
- Drink ten to twelve glasses of pure water a day.
- Eat moderately and deliberately. Do not read or watch television while eating. Emphasize family conversation.
- Eat a maximum of 1,500 calories per day for the entire twenty-one days.
- Employ the thankful heart attitude for your food and health.
- For each of these twenty-one days, visualize yourself getting well and getting or maintaining your ideal body weight and shape.
- Consume 25 percent of your total daily calories at breakfast. Consume 50 percent at lunch and 25 percent of total calories at dinner. (Do not count the two or three healthful snacks.)

Things to Avoid

The following are foods to avoid for a successful detoxification program:

- High-fat dairy products
- White sugar and white flour
- Fried foods and junk food
- Preservatives, salt, aspartame (NutraSweet) and saccharin
- Red meat (especially salt-cured, smoked, nitrate-cured foods like bacon and pepperoni) and chicken (which can be high in fat)
- Coffee and caffeinated teas
- Carbonated beverages, especially colas
- Alcoholic beverages and all forms of tobacco
- Drinking liquids with your meals because they dilute hydrochloric acid; drink liquids one hour before and two hours after meals
- Prolonged periods of direct sun

After-Detox Tips

After you have successfully completed your detoxification and immune system strengthening program, you will not necessarily continue with the above stringent nutritional program. However, you will want to continue a prudent, healthful program to keep you on track. Below are some eating guidelines to remember for healthy living:

- Continue to include high-fiber content in your diet (i.e. fruits, vegetables, whole grains and cereals).
- Choose whole-wheat breads, bran cereals, rice and pasta.
- Consume legumes like beans, lentils and nuts.
- Use low-fat dairy products or dairy substitutes like rice or soy milk.
- Limit your consumption of red meats. Eat chicken or turkey (no skin), tuna and other fish for variety.

- Emphasize fruits, vegetables and salads (with low-calorie dressings).
- Ingest omega-3 fatty acids found in fish oils.
- Drink ten to twelve glasses of purified water per day (instead of carbonated beverages).
- Increase calories back to normal maintenance levels for active individuals (1,800 to 2,400 for females, 2,400 to 3,000 for males) once you achieve your desired weight. To find out your ideal calorie intake, visit a dietician (or www.dietician.com/ibw/ibw.html).

Additives, Metals and Other Toxins

The links connecting heavy toxic metals, food additives or other toxins to poor nutrition are numerous. Toxic metals are commonly found in commercially processed foods that typically contain colorings and additives. Pesticides, herbicides and other agricultural chemicals are often present in our foods as well. The following sections address the problems with metals, food additives and other toxins in the average diet. (For more complete information on this topic, see Dr. Skye Weintraub's *Natural Treatments for ADD and Hyperactivity*, 1997).

Metals

Let's take a look at some of the metals commonly found in the body that become toxic and cause serious degenerative health problems. There are treatment plans available for removing toxic metals from the body, and there are also naturopathic health practitioners who do toxicity testing.

Mercury

Mercury is second only to cadmium as the most toxic heavy

"I feel so empowered and encouraged!"

I cannot thank you enough for the interest and concern you have already shown in my fibromyalgia case. Our telephone conversation amounted to the longest medical consultation I have ever had! I feel so encouraged and empowered to start to return my life to something like normality. Thank you also for arranging with my husband to have all the necessary supplements forwarded to me.

God Bless You.

Sydna

England

metal on earth. Mercury amalgam tooth fillings are one of the primary ways that mercury gets into the body. Some other common places to find mercury include processed foods, drinking water, pesticides, fertilizers, mascara, floor waxes, body powder, adhesives, wood preservatives, batteries and air conditioning filters.

Lead

Lead is linked to a number of neurological and psychological disturbances. Lead has neurotoxic effects on the brain, and our drinking water appears to be one of the more prominent ways we accumulate lead into the body. As a precaution, you should have your water supply tested for high lead levels. Lead-based solders in modern copper plumbing systems increase amounts of lead in our drinking water, so filter your home water supply to remove heavy metals. In addition, always wash your fruits and vegetables in filtered water before use. If possible, buy your produce from farms and areas that have low air pollution. Do not use any imported canned food, as the cans are often lead lined.

Copper

Stress from fibromyalgia can lead to copper toxicity. When the adrenal glands function properly, they produce a copper-bonding protein that rids the body of copper; therefore, stress can deplete zinc from body tissue, which taxes the adrenal glands. People who consume large amounts of soda pop, junk foods and other empty-calorie foods are much more prone to copper toxicity problems, which leads to lowered immune function and recurrent infections.

Manganese

Excessive levels of manganese are toxic to the brain's neurons. There is typically emotional instability associated with manganese overload, such as easy laughter or crying, muscular weakness, slowed speech and impaired equilibrium.

Cadmium

Cadmium levels are typically higher in people that eat excessive amounts of carbohydrates, which suggests that the consumption of fast or refined foods that are low in nutrients increases the body's cadmium levels. Adequate zinc intake may help protect against the adverse effects of cadmium. Once cadmium is in the body it is very difficult to remove because of its seventeen to thirty year life span. Elimination of cadmium from the body is generally accomplished through nutritional therapy.

Cigarettes are a major source of cadmium in our society. Zinc, used for galvanizing iron, can contain up to 2 percent cadmium, and this is one reason our tap water is normally contaminated.

Aluminum

High levels of aluminum affect the central nervous system and are suspected to be intricately involved in the problems of fibromyalgia sufferers. Some of the primary sources of aluminum are in aluminum cookware used in homes and aluminum foil that we frequently use to store food. Aluminum is also found in antacids, bleached flour and coffee. Deficiencies of magnesium and calcium may greatly increase the toxic effects of aluminum in the body.

Food Additives

About 70–80 percent of the foods we consume undergo some degree of refinement or chemical alteration. The Department of National Health and Welfare explains that additives are usually chemical in nature and do not include seasonings, spices or natural flavorings. Consumers in America use approximately 100 million pounds of food additives per year. The FDA in the United States allows more than 10,000 food and chemical additives in our food supply. The average American consumes between ten and fifteen pounds of salt and additives per year (Gans, 1991).

There are two categories of food additives: those that make food more pleasant to the eyes and more appealing to the taste buds and, secondly, those that prevent food from spoiling and increase its shelf life.

BHT

Butylated hydroxytoluene (BHT) retards rancidity in frozen and fresh pork sausage and freeze-dried meats. BHT is also found in shortenings and animal fats, and it is also the base product for chewing gum. Enlargement of the liver and allergic reactions are two of the adverse effects that have been exhibited from the use of BHT.

BHA

Butylated hydroxyanisole (BHA) is also an antioxidant and affects liver and kidney function within human beings. BHA has been associated with behavior problems in children and is commonly used as a preservative in a wide variety of products like baked goods, candy, chewing gum, soup bases, breakfast cereals, shortening, dry mixes for desserts, potatoes, potato flakes and ice cream.

Caffeine

Caffeine can affect blood sugar release and uptake by the liver, and it is a central nervous system, heart and respiratory stimulant. Caffeine is an ingredient in tea, coffee and cola. Some of its ill effects are irregular heartbeat, ear noises, insomnia, irritability and nervousness.

Aspartame

Equal and NutraSweet are brand names of aspartame. Aspartame intensifies the taste of sweeteners and flavors and is about 200 times sweeter than sucrose. Recent research suggests that memory loss attributed to diabetes is caused by aspartame. Large amounts consumed over time will upset neurotransmitter balance and amino acid balance within the body.

MSG

Canned tuna, snack foods, and soups and a large percentage of prepared foods now found on grocery store shelves contain MSG. Monosodium glutamate is now the most common flavor enhancer on the market. It is very difficult to identify MSG on product labels because the manufacturers are not required to call it "MSG" on the label. MSG is very frequently disguised with such names as "sodium caseinate," "hydrolyzed yeast," "hydrolyzed vegetable protein" and "autolyzed yeast." Other names used to disguise MSG are "textured protein," "hydrolyzed protein," "yeast food," "calcium caseinate," "natural chicken [or turkey] flavoring," "yeast extract," "hydrolyzed yeast," "natural flavoring" and "other spices." Side effects of MSG include headaches, numbness, depression, anxiety, heart palpitations and weakness (Elkins, 2001).

Phosphates

Phosphates attract the trace minerals in foods and then continue to remove them from the body causing deficiencies. There are phosphates in cheese, baked goods, carbonated drinks, canned meats, powdered foods and dry cereals. Phosphates are preservatives that prevent the outward chemical changes of food influencing texture, appearance, flavor and color.

Sorbate

Sorbate is a preservative and fungus preventative used in chocolate syrups, drinks, soda fountain syrups, baked goods, deli salads, cheese cake, fresh fruit cocktail, pie fillings, preserves and artificially sweetened jellies.

Sulfites

Sulfites are preservatives and bleaching agents found in sliced fruit, beer, ale and wine. They are commonly found in packaged lemon juice, potatoes, salad dressings, gravies, corn syrup, wine vinegar, avocado dip, and sauces. Sulfites are primarily used to reduce or prevent discoloration of light colored vegetables and fruits such as dehydrated potatoes and dried apples. Sulfites assist vegetables and fruits to look fresh.

8

Natural Supplements and Herbal Remedies

"Your persistence is your belief in yourself."
– BRIAN TRACY

M ore and more physicians are becoming interested in alternative and natural treatments, especially in the treatment of chronic conditions like fibromyalgia. This trend is primarily the result of positive data underscoring the effectiveness of alternative medicine in helping people regain and maintain their health and vitality. At the same time, the conventional physician may not be that knowledgeable about natural treatments because of limited time. The average physician has a hard time keeping up on all the new drugs, let alone study all the breakthroughs on herbs, vitamins, minerals, supplements and nutritional treatments.

People with fibromyalgia and other chronic conditions should use caution when self-treating without the guidance of a physician or health professional who is well trained in nutrition and natural medicine. There are so many products and so much information available that it is easy to be confused about what to use and how to use it. However, with proper guidance, you can be successful in returning to vibrant health and an active lifestyle.

In the last few chapters, I have made a number of supplement recommendations, but this chapter contains a more complete list and description of the minerals, vitamins, herbs and supplements that may be helpful for fibromyalgia and other systemic conditions. Most nutritional supplements treat one or more of the following symptoms: muscle and joint pain, sleep disorders, fatigue, digestive complaints, mental fogginess, depression, headaches, anxiety and a weakened immune system.

Minerals Are Crucial

Decades of research support the essential role of minerals in proper nutrition and health. Minerals are necessary for the healthy development and function of the body, and deficiencies can cause illness and even death. Minerals are absolutely the most important of all the body's nutrients. Even though the body needs only small amounts of many minerals, they need to be supplied on a daily basis to maintain and regulate necessary body functions. Minerals are key because vitamins, amino acids, enzymes, fats and carbohydrates all require minerals for their activity. Without minerals, they cannot be absorbed and utilized.

Minerals are also necessary for normalizing the heartbeat, improving the brain and mental abilities, stabilizing the nervous system, increasing energy and fighting fatigue, balancing electrolyte levels, and assisting the metabolic process. There are eighty-four known minerals, seventeen of those being essential. If there is a shortage of one or more, the balance of the body's systems can be thrown off. One of the vital functions of minerals is that they assist in the regulation of the delicate balance of body fluids. They are vitally important in the process of osmosis, which includes emptying the body of waste and bringing oxygen and nutrients to the cells. In essence, minerals are essential for all mental and physical functions.

More and more people are suffering from mineral deficiencies as minerals continue to disappear from our soils and food supply. Minerals are disappearing from our food supply faster than updated charts can be published. Tables showing the nutrient content of foods can no longer be relied upon because of this fact. There is also a great variation of mineral content of foods because they are being grown under different conditions and in different locations. If minerals are scarce in plants, they are also scarce in human bodies. This appears to be one of the major problems for the fibromyalgia sufferer. After long periods of undue stress and emotional disruption, there is almost always a deficiency of some of the minerals, especially magnesium. Growing evidence supports the fact that stress and anxiety over long periods of time result in mineral imbalances, and this appears to be one of the primary factors that promotes the onset of fibromyalgia. When there is a deficiency of minerals, the result is a nutritional imbalance that can also lead to a disruption of sleep patterns, concentration, and the ability to interact normally (Weintraub, 1997). Mineral-deficient plants also tend to be deficient in vitamins and in protein. It's a known fact that the amino acid component of protein is what forms neurotransmitters and neurotransmitters are vital to mental functioning.

Research is being done on the importance of various minerals, and it now appears that iron and iodine are very important as trace minerals. Chromium, zinc, manganese, magnesium and copper also appear to be essential to good health. The following is a list of the important minerals and their nutritional value for the fibromyalgia sufferer and others with chronic conditions (Tenney, 1995).

Magnesium

Magnesium is a major regulator of cellular activity, including the maintenance of DNA and RNA, and it is considered an anti-stress mineral. Magnesium has a calming effect and is effective

"I began to put your steps into action"

I just wanted to take a moment to thank you so much for your book. I feel as though it has saved me.

My two younger children and I were involved in a car accident two years ago in which all three of us received whiplash. My son, who just turned thirteen, has nodules very badly in his neck and shoulders, though my daughter seems to have recovered very well. I was diagnosed with fibromyalgia after a year and a half of thinking I had become a hypochondriac.

I read about others in your book and identified with them as it seemed that doctor after doctor said they could find nothing wrong with me. One day I mentioned to my chiropractor that the left side of my face was now numb, and he mentioned fibromyalgia. Every doctor I saw after that said that I basically had to learn to live with it with really no solutions except pain medication. I told one doctor that I didn't want to cover up the pain, I wanted to get better. No help from him.

Then my husband was at the bookstore recently and came across your book. He immediately bought it for me and I began to put your steps into action. I was already taking lots of vitamin supplements, but I wasn't taking all the ones you mentioned. I took your vitamins and began using them the way you recommended and in the past two months, I have already felt a huge improvement. I can walk longer, stay active longer, and can handle the pain much better. I still experience a lot of numbness and haven't reached that wonderful sleep yet, but I know in time that it will also happen for me.

I have talked to so many different doctors who have very different ideas regarding fibromyalgia. I love your positive approach. I believe this is what kept me form reaching the depression state. Again, thank you, for your incredible book. God bless you.

Karen S.
Nevada

when taken before bedtime. Magnesium is an essential part of the enzyme system but is poorly assimilated by the body, so it should be taken daily by the fibromyalgia sufferer. A chocolate craving is sometimes indicative of a magnesium deficiency, and deficiencies are very common in times of stress, malabsorption, diarrhea, diabetes and kidney disease. This important mineral assists in the absorption of potassium, calcium, phosphorus, sodium, B-complex vitamins, as well as vitamins C and E. Some of the other symptoms of deficiency are weakness, depression, apprehension, irritability in the nerves and muscles, nausea, vomiting, sensitivity to noise, and muscle cramps and insomnia. Magnesium should be taken with calcium.

Calcium

Calcium is critically essential because it is the most abundant mineral in the body. Most of the calcium in the body is located in the bones and the teeth. It is necessary for the transmission of nerve signals and important for the smooth functioning of the heart muscles and muscular movements of the intestines. It is very important for good health, especially if one has a poor diet, suffers from malabsorption or gets little sunshine. Calcium should be balanced with magnesium for proper nerve function and for a healthy body. Calcium, magnesium and zinc all have a calming effect in the body and are very effective if taken before bedtime to help relax muscles and promote sleep. Vitamins A, C, D and phosphorus are also essential for the efficient functioning of calcium. Some of the symptoms of a calcium deficiency are tingling of the lips, fingers and feet, leg numbness, muscle cramps and sensitivity to noise. (*Note:* Do not take antacids to make up for calcium deficiency.)

Potassium

Potassium is responsible for normal heart and muscle function, normal transmission of nerve impulses and normal growth. It works with sodium to regulate the flow of nutrients in and out of the cells and also helps to stimulate the kidneys, keep the adrenals healthy and maintain heart rhythm. Potassium is vital in stimulating nerve impulses that cause muscle contraction. The symptoms of a potassium deficiency include muscle twitches, weakness and soreness, erratic and/or rapid heartbeats, fatigue, glucose intolerance, nervousness, high cholesterol and insomnia.

Chromium

Chromium is essential for the synthesis of fatty acids and the metabolism of blood sugars for energy. It is also known for increasing the efficiency of insulin in carbohydrate metabolism. Symptoms of a deficiency include weight loss, glucose intolerance and psychological confusion.

Selenium

Selenium is considered an aid to other nutrients, especially vitamin E. It is considered a very powerful antioxidant and needed for immune function, cell membrane integrity and DNA metabolism. Selenium is another mineral considered very important for systemic conditions, as it protects the body from drug and heavy metal (aluminum, cadmium and mercury) toxicity.

Zinc

Zinc is a vital component of enzymes in the brain that repair cells. It is very important for hearing, vision, taste and helps to form skin, hair and nails. Zinc also assists with the absorption of vitamins in the body and is essential for the many enzymes involved in digestion and metabolism. Vitamin A must be present for zinc to be properly absorbed by the body. Symptoms of a deficiency include depression, distorted taste sensation, diarrhea, brittle nails and hair, hair loss, fatigue and memory loss.

Manganese

Manganese is found in many enzymes in the body and assists in the utilization of glucose. It also aids in reproduction and normal functioning of the central nervous system. Manganese is also vital for proper brain function, muscles, nerves and is very important for energy production. Some of the symptoms of a deficiency are nausea, dizziness, muscle coordination problems, strained knees, loss of hearing, slow growth of hair and nails, and low cholesterol.

Phosphorus

Phosphorus and calcium work together and are found mainly in the bones and teeth. Phosphorus levels can be decreased by drinking too much soda pop, a lack of vitamin D and stress. Phosphorus is essential for fibromyalgia sufferers because it helps to produce energy as it aids in the oxidation of carbohydrates. Some of the symptoms of a phosphorus deficiency are a loss of appetite, irregular breathing, nervous disorder, and insomnia.

Iodine

The body requires very little of the trace mineral iodine, but it is essential for the thyroid hormone thyroxine. When supported by iodine, the thyroid gland helps to facilitate energy production. A malfunctioning thyroid can, of course, cause additional symptoms of fatigue and lethargy. Other symptoms of iodine deficiency are swollen fingers and toes, dry hair, cold hands and feet, and irritability. Too much iodine also negatively affects the thyroid gland.

Iron

Iron is a mineral that everyone is very familiar with, yet many people still suffer from an iron deficiency. Iron is not easily absorbed by the body and requires an adequate amount of hydrochloric acid for proper assimilation. Vitamins C and E are also necessary if iron is to be utilized efficiently. Iron is known as the anti-anemia mineral because of its assistance in the oxygenation of cells and combining with protein to form hemoglobin.

Vanadium

There is not a great deal of information available on vanadium, but researchers believe that this trace mineral probably assists in preventing heart disease. Vanadium is a cofactor to insulin and, along with chromium, is very efficient in breaking down fats and sugars, which helps to keep coronary arteries clear. This mineral is vital in the creation of energy.

The Nature of Vitamins

A significant number of people with fibromyalgia and other systemic conditions also suffer from vitamin deficiencies. Vitamins are complex organic substances necessary for life and good health. Vitamins are constantly used in the body and must be replaced daily. They must be obtained from the food we eat and supplements. Vitamins are necessary for the body to utilize other nutrients. Plus, they contribute to breaking down fats, carbohydrates and protein into usable forms.

There are two types of vitamins—fat soluble and water soluble. "Water soluble" means that the vitamin combines with water in the body to function and then is excreted in the urine. Most vitamins fall into the water-soluble category. They only remain in the system for two to three hours, so they must be taken regularly. The fat-soluble vitamins are A, D, K and E. They combine with the fats to be absorbed in the body and remain in the body for a much longer period of time.

Vitamins should normally be taken before meals in order for proper absorption to take place. The following information will be beneficial to the person with fibromyalgia and those with other systemic conditions:

Vitamin A

Remember that vitamin A is a fat-soluble vitamin and can be toxic if taken in large quantities. Beta carotene is nontoxic, however, and is converted to vitamin A in the body on an as-needed basis. This is why one can take up to 25,000 IU of beta carotene on a daily basis without a toxic effect.

Vitamin A helps maintain and repair muscle tissue, treats skin problems, fights infection and aids in the growth and maintenance of healthy bones, skin, teeth and gums. Some good sources of vitamin A are yellow and green vegetables, eggs, milk, liver, fish liver oils, carrots, apricots and sweet potatoes. Some symptoms of a vitamin A deficiency include dry hair, itchy and burning eyes, sinus trouble and fatigue.

Vitamin C (Ascorbic Acid)

Vitamin C is a water-soluble vitamin that is essential to the body. It helps prevent infection by increasing the activity of white blood cells and assists in destroying viruses and bacteria. It also performs as a powerful antioxidant and is considered an anti-stress vitamin. Vitamin C is essential for healing and the synthesis of neurotransmitters in the brain and, when combined with bioflavonoids, also assists with adrenal and immune functions. It helps in the formation of collagen, which is essential for good skin, bones, teeth, and growth in children.

The following conditions usually call for an increase in vitamin C: infections, fevers, injuries, excessive physical activity, anemia and cortisone use. Excellent sources of vitamin C include citrus fruits, cantaloupe, vegetables, broccoli, cauliflower, and red and green peppers. Some herbs that are good vitamin C sources are hawthorne berries, passionflower, olive oil, ginseng and horsetail.

Vitamin E (Tocopherol)

One of the tremendous values of vitamin E for fibromyalgia sufferers is that it assists them in calming down and relaxing. Selenium increases the effectiveness of vitamin E and it is activated by vitamin A. It helps control the unsaturated fats in the body and is thought to reduce cholesterol, helps to normalize brain function, and protects glands during stress. Vitamin E is also considered one of the powerful antioxidants and is needed for cholesterol metabolism, blood clotting, lung metabolism, muscle and nerve maintenance, and body cleansing. Some good sources of vitamin E are peanuts, vegetable oils, lettuce, wheat germs, whole grains, spinach, corn and egg yolks. The herb kelp is also a good source of vitamin E.

B-Complex Vitamins

Fibromyalgia patients need more B vitamins since they are under a great deal of stress, and B vitamins assist in the calming process and good mental health. They are also vital in the production of serotonin, a chemical in the body that influences calming behavior. When B vitamins are deficient, due to inadequate nutrition or increased demand, it can significantly contribute to the lack of an ability to handle stress. B-complex vitamins work together to calm the nervous system and support correct brain function, as well as to improve concentration and memory. Much care should be taken when taking the B vitamins; too much vitamin B6 can cause a folic acid deficiency.

- *Vitamin B1 (Thiamine).* Vitamin B1 is necessary for digestion, blood cell metabolism, muscle metabolism, pain inhibition, and energy. B1 is a water-soluble vitamin and is needed in small amounts on a daily basis. Some good sources of B1 are rice bran, wheat germ, oatmeal, whole wheat, sunflower seeds, brewer's yeast and peanuts. Herbs that contain vitamin B1 are gotu kola, kelp, peppermint, slippery elm and ginseng.

- *Vitamin B2 (Riboflavin).* Vitamin B2 is necessary for antibody formation, red blood cell formation, cell respiration, fat and carbohydrate metabolism. B2 is also water soluble and must be replaced on a daily basis. It is also essential for proper enzyme formation, normal growth and tissue formation. Some good sources of vitamin B2 are wild rice, liver, fish, white beans, sesame seeds, wheat germ and red peppers. A few of the herbs containing B2 are gotu kola, kelp, peppermint and ginseng.

- *Vitamin B3 (Niacinamide).* Vitamin B3 assists the body in producing insulin, female and male hormones, and thyroxine. B3 is also needed for circulation, acid production and histamine activation. Some good sources of vitamin B3 are white meat, avocados, whole wheat, prunes, liver and fish. Symptoms of a B3 deficiency are hypoglycemia, memory loss, irritability, confusion, diarrhea, ringing in the ears, depression and insomnia.

- *Vitamin B6 (Pyridoxine).* Vitamin B6 is helpful in converting fats and proteins into energy, and with the production of red blood cells. It is also essential for proper chemical balance in the body. B6 is especially helpful to the fibromyalgia sufferer who is experiencing excessive stress. Symptoms of a B6 deficiency include irritability, nervousness, depression, muscle weakness, pain, headaches, PMS and stiff joints.

- *Vitamin B12 (Cobalamin)*. Vitamin B12 is essential for iron absorption; fat, protein and carbohydrate metabolism; blood cell formulation; and cell longevity. A strict vegetarian will need B12 supplements. Some symptoms of a B12 deficiency include headaches, memory loss, dizziness, paranoia, muscle weakness, fatigue and depression.

- *Biotin*. Biotin is especially needed if you are under excessive stress, experiencing malabsorption, or have a poor nutrition program. Biotin aids in protein, fat and carbohydrate metabolism, fatty acid production, and cell growth. Some of the symptoms of a biotin deficiency are muscle pain, nausea, anemia, fatigue, high cholesterol and depression.

- *Pantothenic Acid*. Pantothenic acid is needed for the normal functioning of muscle tissue and protects membranes from infection. It is also essential for energy conversion, blood stimulation, and detoxification. Individuals under excessive stress and/or with poor diets need pantothenic acid to assist in normal body functioning. Symptoms of a deficiency include digestive problems, muscle pain, fatigue, depression, irritability and insomnia. Because of the muscle pain, fatigue and depression related to a deficiency of pantothenic acid, supplementation is vital for fibromyalgia sufferers.

- *Para Aminobenzoic Acid (PABA)*. PABA assists in facilitating protein metabolism, promoting growth and blood cell formation. Some of the symptoms of a PABA deficiency are depression, fatigue, irritability, nervousness, constipation and eventually arthritis.

Vitamin P (Bioflavonoids)

Bioflavonoids work together with vitamin C to strengthen connective tissue and capillaries. Bioflavonoids are also essential to assist the body in utilizing most of the other nutrients.

Good sources of bioflavonoids are spinach, cherries, rosehips, citrus fruits, apricots, blackberries and grapes. Herbs that contain bioflavonoids are paprika and rosehips.

Herbal Supplements

Mother Nature provides herbs that have been used by mankind as healing agents since the dawn of history. In ancient times, people were not aware that all the chemical elements contained in the leaves, root, bark, fruits and flowers of herbs are the same chemicals that make up the human body. Modern technology has substantiated the use of herbal medicines and has proven why they have been used successfully for so long. Herbs contain various biochemical constituents—hormones, enzymes, vitamins, minerals, essential fatty acids, chlorophyll, fiber and many other important elements. Herbs provide the body with vitamins, minerals and other nutrients needed to boost the immune system and to aid the body in healing itself.

Herbs are most effective when used in their natural, balanced state. The body appears to be able to utilize herbs when and where they are needed, and naturalists believe the body is readily able to receive and assimilate their nutrients. Herbs are different from drugs in that they almost always contain elements in the amounts that nature intended. Herbalists believe that the natural approach of using herbs can add health and vigor to the body because herbs provide a broad array of catalysts that work together synergistically and harmoniously, resulting in the complete healing of the body in most cases.

Drugs made synthetically from plants are no longer in their natural form, and people often find that these drugs cause more harm than good because of side effects. In contrast, herbs are natural, safe and often do not cause side effects. Still, herbs need to be used with wisdom and knowledge. They should not be used or mixed with other medications unless directed by a physician.

Single herbs do not always contain the proper healing qualities that are required for the symptoms being treated. Herbal combinations, however, are generally formulated to complement one another. By combining several herbs together, formulas are able to treat many symptoms that a single herb cannot. The following is a list of some of the herbs and natural nutrients that may be of benefit to those with fibromyalgia and other systemic conditions.

Red Clover

Red clover is a natural blood purifier and builder and is normally used in its liquid form. It is used to give the body energy and to protect and strengthen the immune system. This herb is high in vitamin A and is an excellent choice in any tea blend since it is usually more effective when complemented with other herbs. Some of the herbs complementary to red clover are prickly ash bark, echinacea, cascara sagrada bark, rosemary and buckthorn bark.

Research has indicated that red clover contains some antibiotic properties that are beneficial against bacteria. This herb has been used for treating bronchitis, cancer and nervous conditions, and for removing toxins from the body. It is invaluable to the fibromyalgia sufferer because it is high in selenium, which is very important in the nutritional regimen, and because it also contains manganese, sodium, calcium, copper, magnesium and B-complex vitamins. Red clover contains vitamin C as well, which is necessary for boosting the immune system and preventing disease.

Passionflower

This herb has properties that are helpful for the nerves and circulation. Passionflower works well in formulas designed to treat insomnia and also works effectively to combat nervous tension, anxiety, stress, restlessness and nervous headaches.

Passionflower is helpful for fevers and is one of the more effective herbs for the nervous system.

Valerian

Valerian is probably the herb most widely used for anxiety and nervous tension. It is used as a natural sedative to improve the quality of sleep and relieve insomnia, and is also used to combat depression. Valerian contains essential oils and alkaloids that reportedly combine to produce its calming, sedative effect. Considered a nervine herb, it is used as a very safe herbal sedative and for after-pains in childbirth, heart palpitations, muscle spasms and arthritis. Valerian is rich in calcium, which accounts for its ability to strengthen the spine, nerves and brain. It is also high in magnesium, which works with calcium for healthy bones and the nervous system, and selenium and manganese to strengthen the immune system, as well as zinc and vitamins A and C.

Chamomile

Chamomile possesses relaxing properties that are very effective in promoting relaxation and inducing sleep. It is also promotes digestion and assists in assimilating nutrients from food, thereby enhancing metabolism and the utilization of energy.

Ancient Egyptians used chamomile for its healing properties. Recent studies have proven chamomile to have antihistaminic effects, along with antiulcer and antibacterial properties. It is useful for cleansing the liver, increasing mental alertness, promoting natural hormones, and for revitalizing the texture of skin and hair.

Chamomile is high in calcium and magnesium, which strengthen the nervous system, promote restful sleep and improve the strength of the immune system. It also contains vitamins A, C, F and B-complex, making it effective for the nervous system. Selenium and zinc, significant for the immune system, are also found in chamomile. Finally, the herb contains tryptophan, the component that allows it to work as a sedative and promote sleep.

Pau d'Arco

Pau d'arco is reported to be a natural blood cleanser and builder. It also possesses antibiotic properties, which aid in destroying viral infections in the body. It helps combat cancer and has been used to strengthen the body, increase energy and strengthen the immune system.

Ginseng

Ginseng is one of the most used herbs in the world. Research has shown that the roots are effective against bronchitis and heart disease. Ginseng has also been found to reduce blood cholesterol, improve brain function and memory, increase physical stamina, stimulate the endocrine glands, strengthen the central nervous system and build the immune system.

Ginseng has been rated as the most potent of herbs because it supports so many body functions. It benefits the heart and circulation, normalizes blood pressure and prevents arteriosclerosis. It is also used to help protect the body against radiation and as an antidote to drugs and toxic chemicals.

Ginseng contains vitamins A and E, components essential for a healthy heart and circulatory system. It also contains the B vitamins thiamine, riboflavin, B12 and niacin, all necessary for maintaining healthy nerves, hair, skin, eyes and muscle tone. The minerals magnesium, iron, calcium, potassium and manganese are also found in ginseng.

Goldenseal

Goldenseal assists in boosting a sluggish glandular system

and promoting hormone production. A very powerful nutrient that goes directly into the blood stream and assists in regulating liver function, goldenseal is reported to act as a natural form of insulin by providing the body with nutrients necessary to produce its own insulin. This aids metabolism and energy production and makes goldenseal a very effective nutrient for fibromyalgia. It is also reported to act as a natural antibiotic to stop infections.

Goldenseal contains the alkaloids hydrastine and hydrastinine that have strong astringent and antiseptic effects on mucus membranes. The antibiotic properties of goldenseal are largely due to its alkaloid content, including berberine, which has been found to be effective against organisms such as *Staphylococcus, Streptococcus, Salmonella* and *Candida albicans*. Goldenseal is a very powerful immune booster. This herb contains vitamins A, C, E, F and B-complex. It also contains potassium, phosphorus, iron, calcium, zinc and manganese.

Gotu Kola

Gotu kola is said to be a valuable treatment for depression because it helps with mental fatigue and memory loss. Naturalists recommend gotu kola for rejuvenating the nervous system. It is sometimes referred to as "brain food" because of its ability to energize brain function. It is also used to increase circulation, neutralize blood toxins, help balance hormones and relax the nerves.

Gotu kola is rich in magnesium and also contains vitamins A, C and K, which protect the lungs from disease and the immune system against diseases. Vitamin K is necessary for blood clotting and in healing colitis. Gotu kola is a good source of manganese, niacin, zinc, calcium, sodium, and vitamins B1 and B2.

Herbal Teas for Fibromyalgia Relief

There are a number of delicious herbal teas that are excellent alternatives to soft drinks and bottled fruit juices that are both normally loaded with sugar. Try herbal teas such as chamomile, spearmint, peppermint, cinnamon, orange peel and valerian root. You can drink the tea hot or chilled, or you can make it into popsicles by pouring it into molds and freezing it. A calming and soothing combination tea for help in inducing sleep is passionflower, valerian, hops and chamomile. Take the tea half an hour before bed. Green herbal teas are especially helpful particularly for strengthening the immune system.

Aloe Vera

Although the aloe vera plant looks like a cactus, it is actually a member of the lily family. Aloe vera is known to promote healing when used externally. It has also been used effectively for treating radiation burns. Also, aloe vera is known to help increase movement in the intestines, promote menstruation, relieve constipation and aid in digestion. In this way, it helps eliminate toxins in the body. Aloe vera has been used very effectively to assist with inflammation and ulcers. It can also help clean, soothe and relieve pain. It contains salicylic acid and magnesium, which function together as an analgesic.

Aloe vera is high in vitamin C and selenium, two powerful antioxidants that help prevent and cure diseases. It also contains vitamins A and B-complex, phosphorus, magnesium, potassium, niacin, manganese and zinc.

Echinacea

Echinacea is a very powerful nutrient that stimulates the immune response in the body and assists the body in increasing its ability to resist infection. It also assists in the promotion of white blood cells and is a blood purifier. Echinacea was used by the Native Americans for snake bites, insect stings and infections.

Echinacea is considered a natural antibiotic. Extracts of echinacea root have been found to contain interferon-like properties. Interferon is produced naturally in the body to prevent viral infections and has been known to fight chemical toxic poisoning in the body.

Echinacea contains vitamin C, which helps to promote healing and fights infections. Calcium and vitamin E are also found in this powerful herb. Echinacea contains iodine, which assists the thyroid gland in regulating metabolism, mental development and energy production. It also contains potassium for muscle contraction, kidney function and nerve function. The sulfur content of echinacea helps to dissolve acids in the body and improve circulation.

Slippery Elm

Slippery elm is a demulcent that buffers against irritations and inflammations of the mucous membranes. A very powerful nutrient for fibromyalgia sufferers, it also helps to assist the activity of the adrenal glands and is a nutritious herb for both internal and external healing. It has been used primarily to treat stomach and intestinal ulcers, gastrointestinal problems, digestion acidity and to lubricate the bowels. Slippery elm is also a blood builder and a supporter of the cardiovascular system.

Slippery elm contains vitamins A, K, F and P—all important in building and toning the lungs, stomach and colon. Minerals contained in slippery elm are selenium, copper, zinc, iron, calcium, phosphorus and potassium. It is equal to oatmeal in vitamin and mineral content.

Rosemary

Rosemary can often replace aspirin for the treatment of headaches. This unique herb assists in combating stress and improving memory. It is very high in calcium and is considered of benefit to the entire nervous system.

Other Supplements

Apple Cider Vinegar

Apple cider vinegar is known as one of the best total body purifiers and cleansers. It is most effective when used in its organic form. It is usually a very potent formula and is best tolerated mixed with a healthy juice or purified water.

Melatonin

In the 1950s, scientists discovered melatonin, a hormone which may be the partial answer to sleep problems. It may also have the capability to affect other common distresses such as lack of immunity, aging and cancer. Melatonin is produced by a small gland found in the center of the brain, the pineal gland. The pineal gland releases melatonin when the eye is not receiving light. Melatonin controls our sleep cycles and helps us to rest soundly. Another tremendous benefit of melatonin is that it contains vitamin E, one of the more powerful antioxidants and free radical fighters.

Malic Acid

Malic acid is a food supplement found in citrus fruits and apples. Studies have found that it assists energy, metabolism and production of muscle energy. When combined with magnesium, malic acid is a very powerful aid for the fibromyalgia sufferer.

Pycnogenol (Proanthocyanadins)

Pycnogenol is a substance produced from grape seed extract and maritime pine bark that has been determined by scientists to be fifty times stronger than vitamin E. Its primary function is that of a very powerful antioxidant that scavenges free radicals generated by foreign toxic chemicals. It has helps remove inflammation from the joints and other tissues, as well as improving the nervous and immune systems. Beyond that, pycnogenol strengthens collagen, improves circulation, enhances the permeability of cell walls, acts as a powerful antioxidant to boost the immune system, enhances metabolism and promotes healing in the body.

Rice Bran Extract

Scientists have found that three of the tocotryonols in the polyphenols of rice bran carry a form of vitamin E that is 6,000 times stronger than current forms of vitamin E. Vitamin E is a powerful antioxidant, immune booster and detoxifier that helps with capillary wall strength, lung metabolism, and muscle and nerve maintenance.

Coenzyme Q10

The discovery of coenzyme Q10 is of tremendous benefit to mankind. It compares with vitamins A, C and E as a powerful antioxidant. Research is supporting the fact that coenzyme Q10 fights diseases associated with nutrient deficiencies such as cancer, aging, heart disease, obesity and fibromyalgia. This nutrient aids in the oxygenation of cells and tissues. It is found in food sources such as spinach, sardines and peanuts. Coenzyme Q10, estimated to be 20 times stronger than vitamin E, is considered to boost biochemical ability and activate cellular energy while improving circulation. One research study found that coenzyme Q10 literally doubled the immune system's ability to clear invading organisms from the blood.

DHEA (Dehydroepiandosterone)

DHEA, an adrenal hormone, is the most abundant hormone in the body and is often considered "the mother hormone." It is a precursor to the sex hormones, as well as a number of other vital hormones in the body. Levels of DHEA are the highest when we are in the prime of life (age 20–35). DHEA is now available without prescription and has great value in preventing and treating osteoporosis, diabetes, cancer, Alzheimer's, cardiovascular disease, high cholesterol and other immune disorders, such as chronic fatigue syndrome and fibromyalgia. It is also thought to be effective in reducing the symptoms of PMS and menopause. It is sometimes called the "miracle" hormone because it is believed to slow down and even reverse the aging process. When recommended nutrients are ingested to boost and balance the bodily systems, DHEA is produced naturally and more readily in the body.

L-Carnitine

L-carnitine is an amino acid that assists greatly in breaking down fats and sugars for energy in the metabolic process. It effectively boosts energy levels in fibromyalgia patients.

Bee Pollen

Bee pollen is very high in protein, and it is considered one of the most complete foods that we can consume. It contains vitamins, minerals, amino acids, proteins, enzymes and fats. It helps when there is a hormone imbalance in the body. Bee pollen is very useful to fibromyalgia patients because it helps to increase appetite, normalize intestinal activity, strengthen capillary walls, offset the effects of drugs and pollutants, and is one of the most powerful immune boosters known to man.

Glucosamine

Glucosamine is the key substance that determines how many proteoglycan (water holding) molecules are formed in cartilage. It is also very effective for improvement in arthritic conditions. In fact, a study conducted by the Vulvodynia Project effectively used glucosamine to reduce sensitivity and pain in soft tissue areas of fibromyalgia patients.

Chondroitin Sulfates

Chondroitin sulfates are naturally occurring substances that inhibit the enzymes that can degrade cartilage. At the same time, it helps to attract fluid to proteoglycan molecules.

9

The Exercise Prescription

*"We are what we repeatedly do. Excellence, then,
is not an act, but a habit."* – ARISTOTLE

In addition to dietary changes and nutrient supplementation, I highly recommend starting an exercise program. Although exercise for fibromyalgics has been a subject of debate, many experts now recommend certain kinds of regular exercise for fibromyalgia sufferers to recover and maintain their health. Regular exercise helps guard against a host of health problems such as obesity, diabetes, high blood pressure and heart disease. It is a proven fact that a lifestyle without exercise is second only to smoking as the most common cause of death in the United States.

At one time it was thought that exercise exacerbated fibromyalgia, but we now know that regular and appropriate exercise is an excellent means of assisting the muscles to become healthy and vibrant. Exercise is one of the key components in a healing regimen for those with existing fibromyalgia. Exercise improves muscle tone by increasing the flow of blood into the tissues. It improves flexibility, increases healing endorphins in the immune system, enhances the production of T cells necessary for an efficient immune system, and stimulates the secretion of serotonin and the growth hormone. As I mentioned in an earlier chapter, imbalances of serotonin and growth hormone have been linked to fibromyalgia.

In fact, the right exercises are essential to weight control, pain reduction and increased mobility in fibromyalgia patients. In a 1989 issue of the *Journal of Hematology*, it was hypothesized that the pain in fibromyalgia is related to microtrauma in deconditioned muscles and that exercise works by conditioning these muscles. Also, in a controlled study on the effects of a cardiovascular training program, researchers concluded that daily gentle low-impact aerobic exercise was of benefit to fibromyalgia symptoms (McCain, 1988). Another outstanding benefit of exercise to the fibromyalgia patient is the improved health of the supportive structures and joints.

At one time scientists thought that exercise actually caused arthritis; however, we now know that regular exercise is an excellent means of keeping joints healthy. The old theory that high-impact exercise such as running and high-impact aerobics could wear out joints has been disproved (Fries, 1994). In fact, it has been documented that regular exercise is strong protection against osteoarthritis (Bunning and Materson, 1991). When you move a joint, as you do in weight resistance exercise or stretching, the nutrient-rich synovial fluid in the cartilage is squeezed out, eliminating some of the waste and buffering free radicals just as if the cartilage were a soggy sponge. Consequently, when that pressure is released the fluid rushes back into the cartilage, nourishing it and keeping it moist and healthy. The movement of fluid in the cartilage is critical to the health of the cartilage. Without it, the cartilage becomes thin and dry, and therefore, more susceptible to deterioration and damage. For this reason, exercise is an outstanding medicine for osteoarthritis and other joint problems. It keeps the nourishing fluid flowing into the afflicted joint and reduces pressure on the joint by strengthening support structures. Having healthier joints and stronger support structures around the musculature is also a tremendous benefit to the fibromyalgia patient. One can also readily see that the right exercise can help to reduce pain and increase the mobility of the fibromyalgia patient.

The Critical Nature of Exercise

If exercise is so necessary for the muscles and joints, why does it often feel so wrong, so painful, for fibromyalgics? The human body is marvelously designed with muscles and joints acting as levers and pulleys to perform an incredible array of activities. However, when we are ill or injured, we have a natural tendency to slow down and stop our normal activities in favor of rest and recovery. Sometimes that is definitely the wisest decision, especially if there is a severe back injury or if fever is involved with an illness. However, when we stop moving, the unused muscle and bone atrophy, or waste away. This is exactly what happens to fibromyalgia sufferers who stop normal activities and cut back on the amount of movement and exercise they are getting. They tend to lose muscle tone and strength, and their flexibility becomes limited. As a result, the fibromyalgia symptoms progress more rapidly.

Although diet and nutritional supplements help to rebuild and keep the body strong, it is very important to continue exercising in order to keep the muscles healthy and flexible. Exercise in many different forms, whether it be calisthenics, stretching, weight resistance, walking, swimming or cycling, is now known to be effective as a most important part of the treatment and healing regimen for fibromyalgia. Exercise fights the debilitating effects of fibromyalgia in the following important ways:

• *Exercise strengthens connective tissue* (ligaments and tendons) while enhancing muscle tone. Strong, well-toned and healthy muscles, tendons and ligaments can support the body and the body's movement much more efficiently and ward off pain.

- *Exercise increases the flexibility* and/or range of motion of muscle tissue. Highly flexible or pliable muscles make movement much more efficient and pleasant, while helping to prevent strains, pulls and tears. Very simple functions such as stooping, sitting, walking and exercising become much easier to perform and much more pleasant. When muscles, ligaments and tendons become more resilient, this means that stiffness will be reduced. Remember that early morning stiffness is one of the major symptoms of fibromyalgia. The resiliency and flexibility that come from exercise also improve the overall muscle and joint function, lessening pain and releasing pent up tensions to aid in stress relief.

- *Exercise increases blood flow to the muscles.* Increased blood flow to muscle tissue enhances the transport of oxygen and nutrients to the muscle fiber, helping to restore and maintain the health of the muscle tissue. We know that people with fibromyalgia do have slightly less blood flow to the muscles, which probably contributes to the pain associated with fibromyalgia. Exercise helps reduce this problem.

- *Exercise increases the body's supply of endorphins.* Endorphins released by the hypothalamus are the body's own morphine-like substance, healing and uplifting with a natural pain-relieving and sleep-deepening effect. Neurologist Norman Harden, M.D., Director of the Pain Clinic at the Rehabilitation Institute of Chicago, supports this theory in his research.

- *Exercise enhances the production of T cells.* It has been validated in research that with exercise, the thymus gland releases a greater abundance of "killer T cells" to boost the immune system and fight foreign cells in the body.

- *Exercise increases levels of serotonin and growth hormone.* Serotonin and growth hormone are the exact pain-reducing and muscle-repair hormones that people with fibromyalgia may lack. Exercise increases their production in the body.

• *Exercise increases the production and flow of synovial fluid* into and out of the cartilage in the joints. The consistent movement of synovial fluid in and out of the cartilage keeps it healthy and well nourished. Healthy joints, of course, are a great benefit to the fibromyalgia sufferer.

As stated earlier, exercise is one of the more beneficial components of the health and healing regimen for the fibromyalgia sufferer. Exercise impacts the individual mentally, physically and emotionally and will:

• tone and strengthen every organ and system of your body.
• relax tension and enhance deep sleep.
• strengthen self-control, increase mental efficiency and enhance feelings of well being and emotional strength.
• help ward off anxiety and depression.
• promote relaxation.
• lower blood fats (triglycerides) and increase good cholesterol (HDLs), thus helping to reduce your risk of coronary heart disease and stroke.
• decrease insulin resistance, aid in the control of blood sugar levels and the treatment of diabetes.
• improve elimination and relieve constipation.
• protect you against osteoporosis and arthritis.
• increase your strength and endurance for both work and play.
• improve your body composition (lowering body fat percent and increasing muscle tissue).
• lengthen your life expectancy.

The Various Areas of Physical Fitness

Understanding the right kinds of exercises for the best health recovery and maintenance program is not as simple as it might sound. Common questions are: How much exercise should I do? When should I do it? Do I walk for heart health or do weight resistance exercises? Do I also have to do stretching and calisthenics? What do I really need do to do for my health and healing regimen?

Given that you already have pain in the muscles as a fibromyalgia sufferer, it would be very wise if you enlisted the service of your medical doctor who can help determine your general level of health and well being. Your doctor, then, can recommend an exercise physiologist or a physical therapist who can help devise the proper exercise program for you based on your current condition with fibromyalgia and your doctor's specifications.

Let's look at areas of exercise and fitness that make up the complete program for both the average person seeking general fitness and the fibromyalgia patient. The three areas of exercise and fitness are cardiovascular fitness, muscular strength, and flexibility.

Cardiovascular Fitness

Cardiovascular fitness refers to your aerobic capacity—the ability of the heart and lungs to supply blood, oxygen and nutrients for vigorous activity. Exercises that increase your cardiovascular fitness also strengthen the joints and improve bone health, therefore preventing osteoporosis.

Exercise aids in weight control, prevents heart disease and lowers high blood pressure. Examples of cardiovascular fitness or aerobic type activities are brisk walking, biking, jogging, stair climbing, swimming, rowing, line dancing and sports that involve continuous movement. Your goal should be to get your heart rate in your target zone and keep it there for at least twenty to twenty-five minutes consistently. (The formula for computing your personalized target heart rate will be provided in the walking section of this chapter.) The key here is finding

"I am able to golf nine holes and enjoy my housework"

I was diagnosed with fibromyalgia about five years ago. I now realize I have had this condition for many years. It was getting to the point where I could no longer go for my long walks, which I loved doing. Climbing stairs, housework, and yard work became extremely difficult. Nothing I tried or was prescribed helped me.

I saw Dr. Elrod being interviewed on our local television station. I ordered a copy of your book and read it. I decided I had to try this formula to see what it would do for me. It will be three years in May 2001 that I have been on your supplements and following your program.

I really feel it is reversing my condition. I am able to go for my five-mile walks again, go hiking on holidays, golf nine holes and do my housework and yard work and enjoy it. My sleeping is much better and I would say my condition has improved 80 percent, although I do try to not overdo anything. My bad days now, which are not near as often, are like my good days before I started your program.

I am truly thankful for your program and what it has done for me.

Diane A.
Canada

the right activity and determining the level at which you can perform it. For example, depending upon the severity of your condition, you may need to begin with gentle walking on a treadmill or riding a stationary bike for only five to ten minutes per session. You can start doing this three to four days per week and gradually increase over several weeks, working up to twenty-five to thirty minute sessions for four to five days per week.

Muscular Strength

Muscular strength is very important for preventing injuries while lifting, doing housework, participating in recreational activities and exercising. Strength training is also called "resistance training" and involves repeatedly lifting a weight or moving against a resistance. Lifting free weights like dumb bells or barbells, or using weight machines and resistance devices like elastic tubing are all examples of resistance exercises.

You do not have to lift several hundred pounds to improve your strength. In fact, depending upon the severity of your condition, you may need to start with three to five pound weights or an equivalent resistance with an elastic tubing device, but the important thing is to get started at an appropriate, comfortable level and progress gradually. I would strongly recommend beginning your exercises with dumb bells (small weights that can be held in one hand), weight machines or elastic tubing devices. These are much easier to work with and much safer than the larger, heavier free weights. Once you have significantly progressed and improved strength, then you can try heavier free weights.

Flexibility

Excellent flexibility is very important because relative muscle inflexibility can cause excessive stress and force to be exerted on areas of the body opposite of the movement. This can very easily lead to injury and worsen the fibromyalgia condition. All types of movement, aerobic activities, as well as strength development activities, can improve flexibility. However, some of the best flexibility exercises are yoga, various martial art forms, and all types of stretching. The more effective and efficient flexibility exercises utilize stretch devices such as elastic tubing. The elastic tubing devices are especially effective because generally you can include both strength development and flexibility movement.

Establishing Your Exercise Program

I believe that muscle strengthening, cardiovascular and stretching exercises can be performed safely and effectively by most fibromyalgia sufferers. Remember that common sense and moderation are always the rules when beginning an exercise program. Be certain that you contact your physician for a thorough examination, and then consult with an exercise physiologist or physical therapist to assist you in tailoring an exercise program for your specific personal needs (and limitations). Remember, if you have an acute flare-up of your condition, your doctor or exercise physiologist might suggest that you restrict your exercises to a stationary bike and very low-impact movement. You may even stop exercising for a short period of time until you can recover to the point that you can effectively begin again.

Beware of personal trainers who mean well but are not familiar with your condition and do not have formal training in designing programs for people with limitations. Also the programs in exercise books should be avoided if they are meant for healthy individuals until your fibromyalgia is completely reversed. A doctor, preferably a rheumatologist who has knowledge of fibromyalgia, should probably devise an exercise program for you following your physician's specifications.

Your health and healing exercise program should be designed so that you are gradually building up muscle and doing more intense exercise for longer periods of time without straining or forcing the point of injury (or causing undue pain). The program should include cardiovascular fitness, muscular strength and muscular flexibility. The following are some guidelines to keep in mind as you proceed with your program:

- *Listen to your body.* Whenever you feel dizzy, become nauseated, experience an undue shortness of breath or feel any pain in the body (especially the chest), then always stop your exercise immediately.

- *Be sure that you avoid doing too much* too soon so that you might avoid unnecessary injury. Remember there is a marked difference between pushing just a little more to improve and pushing yourself to the point of injury. Learn the difference between the two.

- *Learn to establish* the difference between slight muscle soreness due to past workouts and aggravation of fibromyalgia pain.

- *When beginning your exercise program,* remember to go easy and to work at a comfort level, building gradually. Just remember that your body will adapt naturally. You will be amazed at how quickly and readily you will improve and be able to increase resistance and time.

- *Always warm-up carefully*, taking time to create blood flow and increased body heat in the muscle fiber. A proper warm-up will insure a comfortable, enjoyable workout and help you to avoid unnecessary injury.

- *A good rule of thumb* is to always cool down gradually after exercising, and don't abruptly. Bring the heart rate and body temperature down gradually. A good way to cool down is to walk easily, stretch and shake out your arms and legs. The proper cool-down will assist in dissipating lactic acid and will decrease the amount of muscle soreness. You will recover faster and be more refreshed for your exercise the next day.

Effective Exercises

Cardiovascular activity, stretching and weight resistance exercises using elastic tubing devices are the three most effective approaches to health improvement for most fibromyalgia sufferers. Weight training is the area we want to be most careful with. You may decide to start a weight training program only after making improvements in the other two areas. Below are some specific exercises listed with suggested guidelines for performing them safely.

Walking

Walking is one of the most complete, convenient, effective, and enjoyable ways to lose weight and restore or maintain total health. Not only does walking burn calories and fat, it also tones and strengthens muscles, boosts energy, and improves total health and well being. Walking improves muscle flexibility, helps to eliminate early morning stiffness, alleviates muscle pain and improves the overall muscle physiology for energy production—all major problems for the fibromyalgia sufferer.

There are some very important guidelines for you to follow to move you safely and efficiently toward your goal of health and healing. The most effective program combines the proper walking routine along with lifestyle changes like improved nutrition. The most effective way to burn the most calories and to lose weight healthily and efficiently is to walk for a longer time and greater distances as opposed to walking faster and going shorter distances. If time and distance are a problem in the beginning because of a lack of physical condition or obesity, begin with moderate times and distances. For instance, take ten-, fifteen-, or twenty-minute walks initially. After a couple of weeks, do these short walks more than once a day until you can gradually increase your time to thirty to forty-five minutes of continuous walking.

For best results, you should be performing within your target heart rate zone, which is somewhere between 50 percent and 70 percent of your maximum heart rate. To compute your target heart rate (THR), subtract your age from 220 and then subtract your resting heart rate (RHR); multiply by .5 and then add your resting heart rate back into the figure. The formula is as follows:

$$(220 - \text{Age} - \text{RHR}) \times 0.5 + \text{RHR} = \text{THR}$$

For instance, if you are 40 years of age, with a RHR of 65, your most efficient THR for weight loss is 123:

$$(220 - 40 - 65) \times 0.5 + 65 = 123$$

Walking and exercising within this heart rate range, you are giving yourself the best opportunity to walk extended periods without tiring, while still efficiently losing weight and maintaining a state of health. Following this program consistently will assist you in logging twenty to thirty miles per week for a weekly energy expenditure of approximately 2,000–3,000 calories. If you will maintain this program consistently, you can burn just under a pound of fat per week or thirty-five to fifty pounds a year. This can be computed very easily because approximately 3,500 calories equals one pound.

The following are some tips to help ensure your success in your health restoring and walking program:

- *Strive for increased energy and movement,* and positive experiences. Build your health-restoring program around exercise, energy and positive thinking, and it will help to enhance your success. Very often, when we build restoring health and weight loss around food there is a tendency to think only about food. Walking for restored health works not only physiologically, but also has a very strong impact psychologically. It begins to help restore self-esteem, it energizes and raises our metabolism.

- *Think consistency and make a commitment.* If you made the commitment to do what is necessary on a daily basis with lifestyle changes to restore your health and vitality, then you are on your way to success. Writing your goals down will help to insure your success. (There are suggestions in Chapter 4 that will help you in the goal setting process.)

- *Walk six days a week.* You may read that three days a week is sufficient for good heart health. That may be true if you are only working toward maintaining good heart health, but remember you have made a commitment to restore your health. You have to be consistent with your lifestyle change in order to overcome the symptoms and conditions of fibromyalgia. If you set a goal to walk only three days a week, it might become too easy to get away from your program by missing too many days. If you walk six out of seven days, on the other hand, it becomes part of your lifestyle. It becomes a habit and you will look forward to it. If you take a break and have one day per week off, you'll be more refreshed and then you will look forward to getting back to exercising on the following day.

- *Exercise time and distance are the keys.* To burn more calories, to maintain a healthful weight and to restore good health, the key is to walk consistently—go farther and not faster. Depending on the severity of your condition, you may need to begin with several brief walks daily, even as short as three five-minute walks each day. Then you build up gradually, so that your pace is comfortable and you do not lose the enjoyment of your walk as you gain benefits. The goal is to work up to the point that you are walking six days per week at your median pace for at least thirty to forty-five minutes per day, burning maximum calories.

- *Don't get hung up on numbers.* Especially early in your exercise program, don't worry about inches and pounds. Simply focus on enjoying your daily exercise regimen. Begin to look forward to it; be consistent and stick with it. If you begin to focus on whether or not your are losing inches and pounds—especially early in a program—it can become very discouraging.

- *Warm up properly for walking.* Do not stretch. You never stretch a cold muscle. The best way to warm up for walking is an easy, gentle walk for the first few minutes to increase blood flow and body temperature gradually. Then increase your walking pace gradually over a period of five or six minutes to a median pace at which you will complete your entire walk. Some experts even recommend adding a few short (one-minute) bursts of increased activity every five to ten minutes to boost your metabolism, but do not strain or overwork yourself. However, if you want to do a few gentle arm circles, body twists and neck rolls to increase blood flow, raise body temperature gradually and gently loosen muscles, ligaments and tendons, feel free to do so for five or six minutes before beginning your gentle warm up walk. After you have completed your walk, then stretch for flexibility.

- *Shoes and clothes are important.* Wear loose-fitting, comfortable clothes and light colors if the heat is severe. Walk in the early mornings and late evenings to avoid extreme heat and humidity. Shoes with good support are very important. Do not walk in old shoes that have been broken down or lost their flexibility. A good running shoe is ideal for the support for joints, ligaments and tendons that you need for efficient walking.

- *Find flat solid surfaces to walk on.* One of the most pleasant places to walk is in your own neighborhood where you have a flat, smooth, asphalt surface, trees and pleasant surroundings. Other good choices are malls, park trails and jogging tracks.

- *Consult your physician before starting a program.* As always, consult your physician before beginning any aspect of an exercise program. For instance, if you have any severe orthopedic problems—for instance, pain in the hip, knee, ankle or another weight-bearing joint, then walking may not be the best exercise for you until those conditions are corrected. Two alternatives are water exercises and cycling.

In summary, a few of the very important benefits of walking are stronger, more flexible muscles, ligaments and tendons, especially in the hips, lower limbs and the lower back. The arms, shoulders and upper back will benefit as well. Strength and flexibility improvement will enhance the physiology of the muscles, therefore, reducing early morning stiffness and alleviating the pain suffered by fibromyalgia victims. Another benefit is that of improved self image and overall sense of well being. Improved cardiovascular fitness will improve stamina and endurance, decrease body fat and increase lean body tissue, which will boost metabolism. Exercise will also decrease heart disease and blood pressure risk, and reduce stress and tension.

Aquatics

Swimming and water exercises are very advantageous to many chronic conditions and are extremely popular with physical therapists, exercise physiologists, and physicians. Patients also enjoy aquatic exercises for the benefits that they normally gain without joint strain. However, I should initially point out that the fibromyalgia patient should proceed with extreme care as water resistance sometimes can equal the weight resistance you may encounter with serious weight-lifting exercises. Those with severe fibromyalgia conditions should proceed very cautiously and under the direction of a professional as vigorous activity or movement in water could worsen the fibromyalgia condition.

Water therapy can be most beneficial, however, especially in heated pools. Also, all three types of exercise that are very important to the fibromyalgia sufferer—strength, flexibility and aerobic—can be accomplished in the water. Just remember that all movement should be very low impact and therapeutic in nature so as not to worsen the fibromyalgia condition.

Another advantage of aquatic activities and exercises is that they can be performed in shallow water or with flotation devices, therefore, not requiring the participants to be expert swimmers. They need not have any swimming experience at all. The following is a list of the benefits derived from aquatic activities and exercises:

- The water provides stability and support, which could be especially beneficial for a fibromyalgia sufferer who has an advanced or extreme condition.
- The therapeutic movements in the water help to relieve stress and anxiety.
- Water exercises promote muscle relaxation, therefore, enhancing relief of pain.
- Stronger, more flexible muscles result from these activities.
- Aquatic exercise is easier on the joints, and healthier joints aid both fibromyalgia and the arthritic patients.
- When participating with a group, the social interaction serves as a tremendous benefit in gaining emotional confidence and developing sociability. It gives fibromyalgics a support group outside of family and friends.
- Aquatic exercises may help boost confidence.
- Water exercise improve heart health and lung capacity, which enhances the health and healing of the entire body.
- Water exercise also builds more strength and flexibility at the muscle/connective tissue junction where the seat of the fibromyalgia problem usually rests.
- Water exercise may also increase serotonin and the growth hormone levels, which will benefit the fibromyalgia condition tremendously.
- The stimulation of the production of T cells strengthens the immune system and boosts the body's ability to heal itself.

Understand that walking and stretching are the two most beneficial types of exercise, especially when strength exercises can be combined with the stretching. However, aquatic exercises are an excellent alternative and can deliver many benefits. If you have access to a pool, especially a heated pool, this is an excellent alternative to your walking and strength/flexibility exercises.

Cycling

Most people with fibromyalgia usually walk for their exercise. However, if you have a very chronic and severe condition with a great deal of pain around the knees and in the hip joints, cycling could be an excellent alternative. Cycling takes weight off of the legs and hips because they are not responsible for supporting your weight while exercising. Cycling may also be ideal for those who have lower back pain, and pain around the knees. Cycling is also something that most everyone already knows how to do, and there is the convenience of cycling either in the neighborhood or on a stationary bike.

Cycling is a tremendous heart and lung conditioner, and also strengthens the quadriceps (the thigh muscles) more than walking. These are the muscles that get you up stairs, assist you in lifting, and get you out of chairs. Cycling exercises also strengthen the muscles around the knee joints, which will greatly reduce the pain areas around the knees. Cycling can provide you with countless health benefits if you adhere to the following guidelines when cycling:

- *Always warm up before every activity,* even cycling. Remember not to warm up by stretching. Do not stretch cold muscles. Warm up with gentle, low–impact body movements and/or easy walking or easy cycling without resistance on a stationary bike or on flat surfaces outside. This will gradually raise the body temperature and increase blood flow.

- *If there is pain in the lower back and the knees,* be sure not to add very much resistance at all in the beginning on a stationary bike and avoid hills and strenuous areas cycling outside. Do this until the legs, heart and lungs become better conditioned, and the pain feels much improved.

- *The bicycle seat should be adjusted* so that your leg nearly straightens when the pedal is at the bottom of the rotation.

This adjustment allows the greatest benefit for muscular development and cardiovascular efficiency.

- *Remember to build up your time and distance* on a gradual basis so as not to aggravate your fibromyalgia condition. You will know as you listen to your body when you can add speed, distance or resistance. With all other aspects of your program, be certain to discuss this with your physician and proceed with his or her approval.

Stretching

Stretching is a vital part of any exercise program for those people with fibromyalgia. Sedentary living habits and increased inactivity are major contributors to the loss of flexibility. Fibromyalgia patients typically adopt more sedentary living habits and become more inactive than normal because of the pain and lack of energy that are usually associated with the condition. This inactivity causes muscles and connective tissue to lose their pliability and allows body fat to increase tremendously, and contributes to decreased flexibility.

Most people tend to lack flexibility in the front of the hip or the back of the thigh, in the lower back, and the neck and shoulders. In order to increase overall body flexibility it is necessary to engage in basic flexibility exercises for the large muscle groups of these areas. If stretching exercises are done properly, there are tremendous benefits for the fibromyalgia patient. However, if done incorrectly, they can do more harm than good and possibly even cause damage. The following are some guidelines to ensure that you get maximum benefit from your flexibility program:

- *You must stretch on a daily basis,* in order to derive the most benefit from your flexibility program. Make a commitment, do it consistently and do it properly. Remember it takes time to make progress, so be patient. Stretching is ideally done after your exercise session.

- *Never use stretching for your warm-up.* Always warm-up before beginning stretching. For instance, do some mild walking and mild calisthenics such as arm swings and body rotations to increase the blood flow and body temperature. Ideally, you should break a sweat before beginning to stretch.

- *Get in the correct, comfortable position* to begin your stretch. Slowly and gently stretch the muscle or muscle group with which you are working. Avoid sudden, bouncing movements because this stimulates sensory receptors that shorten the muscle, which is counterproductive since the muscle you are attempting to stretch is now shorter. When the muscle is stretched slowly and gently, other sensory receptors are activated that override the initial stretch response and prevent muscle contraction. The muscle will relax and you can lengthen it without stress or strain.

  In the beginning, put a very gentle stretch on the muscle, making sure not to feel pain. After holding this gentle stretch position for five to six seconds, the muscle will seem to relax even more (this is called "proprioceptive neuromuscular facilitation"). Once you have stretched just a bit farther, gently and with ease, hold the complete stretch for about ten seconds, and then release it very gently and move slowly back to the original position making sure not to release rapidly.

- *Be careful to select very simple exercises* to begin your stretching program. Some suggested exercises will be given at the end of this section.

- *Remember to concentrate on relaxing* the muscle being stretched, even as it is being stretched. This will facilitate a more efficient, more comfortable, safer stretch. Stretching exercises are not meant to be competitive. Avoid bouncing movements and strenuous stretches. When you feel pain that means you are overstretching and you are possibly inflicting damage to the muscle.

- *Stretching progress will come very slowly.* Don't push or be overanxious.

Stretches for Fibromyalgia Sufferers

The muscle groups that fibromyalgia patients should concentrate on are the arms, shoulders, neck, upper and lower back, hips and the thighs, especially the hamstrings in the back of the thighs. The following stretches will improve joint health and positively impact most of the major fibromyalgia pain centers.

1. *The lower back and buttocks.* Lie on the floor, hands by your side, legs straight and feet together. When lying or sitting for stretches, it is best to perform them on carpet or an exercise pad. Slowly bring both knees toward the chest reaching with your hands just under the knees and pull them toward the chest, bringing both knees as near the chest as possible with a gentle stretch on the lower back and buttocks. Hold for four to five seconds, then try and stretch just a bit farther. Hold for about ten additional seconds in the stretch position, relaxing the muscles that are being stretched as much as possible, then return slowly and gently back to the starting position. Take caution not to strain or put weight on the back of your neck. Resting momentarily between each stretch, perform the movement three to four times. This stretch will affect the pain-sensitive points in the lower back and the center of the buttocks.

2. *The hip extensor and lower back.* Lying on your back, extend your arms straight out to the side with hands at the shoulder level. Raise the left leg up to a vertical position, keeping the leg straight, then twist the body to place your

left foot over across the top of the body attempting to touch the right hand. If you cannot place the left foot into the right hand on the floor, then move the hand to meet the foot. Gently stretch for four to five seconds, and then as you relax the muscle you should be able to extend the stretch a bit farther for the ten-second count. Return to the starting position and repeat on the opposite side. Bring the right foot up to a vertical position, twist body to the left and bring the right foot over and across the body into the left hand for the same count. Perform three stretches on either side while keeping trunk and arms on the mat.

3. *Hip flexors, hamstrings (the back of the thighs) and the lower back muscles.* Lying on your back with hands to side and legs fully extended with feet together, bring left knee toward the chest while keeping the right leg extended, reaching with both hands underneath the knee and pull toward the chest for a gentle stretch position. Hold for the ten-second count and return slowly to the starting position. Repeat the movement with the opposite leg.

4. *The trunk rotators, neck, shoulder and upper back muscles.* Sit on the carpet or the exercise pad, cross both legs with feet pulled as near the buttocks as possible. Keeping body erect, twist to the right, moving both arms, head and neck with the trunk. With trunk, head and neck rotated 90 degrees to the right, reach with right hand and grab upper left arm and pull arm and shoulder gently across the body increasing the stretch on the upper arm, shoulder and upper back. Hold for the ten-second count and return slowly and easily to the starting position. Now repeat the same movement, twisting the trunk to the left, reaching with the left hand, grabbing the upper right arm and pulling it gently across the body for the ten-second count. This stretch is impacting the pain sensitive points in the upper back, over the shoulder blades, and the top of the shoulders and in the lower back.

5. *The lower back and neck muscles.* Sitting with legs crossed and feet as near to the buttocks as possible, keep your upper body straight and erect for the beginning position. Fold arms and bend gently forward attempting to touch the forehead where the legs are crossed in front of the body. Hold a gentle stretch for eight to ten seconds, then return easily and gently to the starting position. Repeat the exercise three to four times. Be cautious not to bounce or strain. The movement should be steady and gentle.

6. *The hamstrings (the back of the thighs), the buttocks and the lower back.* Sit on the floor with legs straight, body erect and feet together. Keeping legs straight, slowly and gently reach forward with both arms putting a gentle stretch on the back of the thighs, the buttocks and the lower back. Reach as far as possible with both hands together and hold for the ten-second count, then return slowly and gently to the starting position. Repeat the movement for three or four repetitions.

7. *The pectoral muscles (the chest), the upper back and the neck muscles.* Starting position is standing directly behind a chair, reaching both hands to the top of the back of the chair and standing far enough away that the upper body is parallel to the floor. Keeping the body and arms straight, perform a gentle stretch from the lower back, bending the body toward the floor, moving the head down between the arms, holding on to the back of the chair, keeping the legs straight. While in the stretch position, move the head down farther, looking back toward the legs, with the head between the arms, placing a gentle stretch on the back of the neck muscles. Hold for the ten-second count, and move easily and gently back to the starting position. Perform four repetitions of the movement.

> ## "I have a new lease on life!"
>
> Thank you for giving me hope. Three days ago I started your program and the pain in my left arm has gone away completely. My body no longer feels stiff all over. I have a new lease on life!
> *Cantor*
> Tennessee

Strength Training

The best devices for strength training are resistance devices like elastic tubing with anchors that can be attached to doors or walls. Less desirable devices for the fibromyalgia patient would be free weights (dumb bells and barbells) or weight machines. These can be used successfully if you work with weights as light as three to five pounds and get professional help for proper exercise regimens and techniques. Still, the most highly recommended weight resistance exercises are those that use elastic tubing. Exercises using elastic tubing are low resistance, flexible and very low impact.

A tremendous advantage of the elastic tubing devices is that strength and flexibility movements are combined within the one device (Elrod, 1996). See the Resource Guide in the back of this book for information on my Body Advantage system.

"Sticking with" Your Program

The key to sticking with your exercise program is to find exercises and a regimen or routine that you thoroughly enjoy. Develop a very positive attitude toward changing your lifestyle and toward exercise in general. Remember that it will be a key component in restoring your health and vitality. Experiment until you find the exercises and the situation that fit you. If you enjoy the water, then join a water exercise or swimming class. If you love the outdoors, then develop exercise regimens and routines outside. If you prefer to be inside, then develop a regimen and routine using exercise equipment, exercise cycles or join a dance class. Use the buddy system—exercise with a family member or a friend. Read or listen to music while you are exercising. Change your routine for variety. There are exercise regimens and routines that are perfect for you, so make them as pleasant and enjoyable as you possibly can and just do it!

Here are some more tips for exercise success:

- *Begin with a positive attitude.* The human mind is a fascinating organism. If you begin with negative thoughts and statements, soon you will succumb to negativism. On the contrary, if you begin with positive attitudes and positive thinking you will purely and simply get positive results.

- *Begin properly.* Obtain professional help to be assured that you can begin your program safely and effectively. A large percentage of those who begin on their own do too much too soon and possibly do more harm than good.

- *Organize and prioritize your daily activities.* Many conclude that "there are not enough hours in the day" or "I would love to, but I just simply do not have enough time." Simply set aside the time, making it a necessary and very important part of your lifestyle. Remember that it is one of the key components of your return to health and vitality.

- *Make it convenient and enjoyable.* Avoid cumbersome routines. Create workout areas right at home and mark off walking tracks and distances right in the neighborhood or nearby parks with pleasant, enjoyable surroundings.

- *Find your time of day.* Find the time of day that you function more efficiently and that works into your schedule most conveniently.

- *Vary your routine.* Do cross- or seasonal training. This helps to prevent boredom and keeps you energized about your program. Cross-training means that you are trying different activities like swimming, walking or cycling. Change your routes or scenery while cycling or walking.

- *Back off on days that you're not quite feeling up to it.* Some days you just might not feel quite up to it so back off and reduce your workout time. Remember that "something is better than nothing." However, some days you might just want to reward yourself. Read a book, paint a picture or go to a movie so that you continue to be motivated for your exercise routine.

- *Keep records and set goals.* A great incentive builder is to keep records of your program involvement. Maintain an interest in keeping up with what you do, how often you do it, your progress, your personal comments and results. Some individuals enjoy taking body measurements, keeping up with blood pressure, change in resting heart rate, etc. Set some goals in these areas and keep up with those with which you have the greatest interest. (See daily log in Appendix B.)

- *Buy new shoes and clothes.* Maintain a reasonable budget, but reward yourself with walking and exercise shorts and clothes that are attractive, comfortable and motivating. Devices such as walkmans and heart rate monitors can also be enjoyable and motivating.

- *Utilize the buddy system.* If you have a workout partner to join you and encourage you on a daily basis, this can help tremendously. Someone waiting for you will stimulate you to exercise on a more regular basis. Enjoying the company and conversation of a good friend or workout partner is something that keeps many people going with the program.

Exercise for Restored Health

I advise all chronic pain sufferers to begin with gentle exercises such as easy stretches, slow low-impact walking, leisurely swimming or light resistance exercises with elastic devices. By all means, get your physician's approval before starting any exercise program. Avoid activities that place abnormal stress on your muscles or joints and cause undue pain. The most critical thing to do is simply start exercising!

10

Coping with Stress and Depression

"In a full heart there is room for everything, and in an empty heart there is room for nothing." – ANTONIO PORCHIA

I cannot talk about fibromyalgia without talking about stress and depression. The effects of these two conditions may not only trigger fibromyalgia, but also perpetuate it. Proper stress (and depression) management are so important for fibromyalics, I decided to dedicate an entire chapter to methods of coping with these dangerous and potentially debilitating diseases.

Typically, anything that limits mobility, threatens disability, or produces pain can lead to increased stress and eventually to a state of depression. This in turn can result in fatigue, a lack of interest in family, friends and sexual activities, as well as many other problems. In fact, depression is a common side effect of fibromyalgia. It is a very natural response to be upset and stressed when pain forces one to give up favorite activities, makes routine chores difficult and constantly reminds one of its presence. The risk of depression increases greatly as the threat of disability becomes apparent and as pain becomes more severe. When unpredictable pain flare ups occur, the fibromyalgia victim tends to feel continuously threatened by the disease.

Handling Stress

Effective stress relief techniques can greatly assist the fibromyalgia patient in fighting (and preventing) depression. Recognize that stress is the response of the mind, body and emotions to everyday happenings and the pressures of life. It is important to understand that stress is not the actual event, but rather our interpretation or emotional reaction to the event. For example, a very active person might find a stress fracture injury very traumatic, while the next person may find it an opportunity to rest up and refresh the body while recovering. The situations are very similar, but it's how the individuals respond to the situation that determines the stress impact (O'Koon, 1996).

This explanation helps explain why some people become much more stressed by the pain, fatigue and other circumstances associated with fibromyalgia than do others. However, even among those that cope with fibromyalgia extremely well, it can still become a very stressful situation. The following are symptoms that will help you to know when you are overly stressed (Dexter & Brandt, 1994):

- irritability
- fatigue
- nervousness
- sweaty, clammy hand

- anxiety
- muscle tension
- nausea
- loss of appetite

Being overly stressed may eventually lead to depression if not managed properly. Also, chronic stress seems to signal certain neurotransmitters to release chemicals that shock the body and weaken the immune system, thus making the fibromyalgia symptoms and circumstances worse and increasing the risk for other conditions and diseases.

In the 1920s, Dr. Hans Selye at the University of Prague did pioneering research demonstrating that emotions can cause illness (Simonton, Simonton, & Creighton, 1992). Dr. Selye's research has since been supported in some more recent studies utilizing both laboratory animals and humans. Many of these studies have also begun to reveal the physiological process by which undue emotional responses or chronic stress can create a susceptibility to disease.

The body is designed so that moments of stress, followed by a physical reaction or release of that stress, will allow little harm; in fact, proper amounts of stress are healthy. However, when the physiological response to stress is not discharged, there is a negative cumulative effect on the body, referred to as chronic stress. Chronic stress is increasingly recognized as a highly significant factor influencing conditions such as fibromyalgia. Dr. Selye has also discovered that chronic stress suppresses the immune system, responsible for controlling cancerous cells and other dangerous microorganisms such as free radicals.

The correlation between health and stress is obvious—in fact, the majority of fibromyalgia victims I have worked with have experienced a traumatic experience which caused a long period of undue or chronic stress in their lives. Interestingly, current research appears to be establishing links connecting traumatic experiences, chronic stress and fibromyalgia. According to research and the observations of various physicians, it appears that disease is more likely to occur following highly stressful events. It has been documented by physicians that when their patients suffered major emotional upsets there is generally an increase, not only in diseases usually acknowledged to be susceptible to emotional influence, (i.e., high blood pressure, obesity, ulcers, headaches), but also in infectious diseases, backaches and even accidents.

Dr. Thomas H. Holmes and his associates at the University of Washington School of Medicine undertook research to validate these observations. They set out to develop a process by which they could objectively measure the amount of stress or emotional upset in an individual's life. The doctors designed a scale that listed traumatic or highly stressful events along with

Social Readjustment Rating Scale

Event	Value
Death of a spouse	100
Divorce	73
Marital separation	65
Jail term	63
Death of a close family member	63
Personal injury or illness	53
Marriage	50
Fired from work	47
Marital reconciliation	45
Retirement	45
Change in family member's health	44
Pregnancy	40
Sex difficulties	39
Addition to family	39
Business readjustment	39
Change in financial status	38
Death of close friend	37
Change to different line of work	36
Change in # of marital arguments	36
Mortgage or loan over $10,000	31
Foreclosure of mortgage or loan	30
Change in work responsibilities	29
Son or daughter leaving home	29
Trouble with in-laws	29
Outstanding personal achievement	28
Spouse begins or stops work	26
Starting or finishing school	26
Change in living conditions	25
Revision of personal habits	24
Trouble with boss	23
Change in work hours, conditions	20
Change in residence	20

Change in schools	20
Change in recreational habits	19
Change in church activities	19
Change in social activities	18
Mortgage or loan under $10,000	17
Change in sleeping habits	16
Change in number of family gatherings	15
Change in eating habits	15
Vacation	13
Christmas season	12
Minor violation of law	11

numerical values. The scale they developed is in the accompanying sidebar "Social Readjustment Rating Scale" (Simonton, Simonton, & Creighton, 1992).

You may have noticed that this scale includes highly stressful events as well as what would be perceived as happy events, such as marriage and promotions. Even though you may be experiencing a number of positive experiences, they still demand a great deal of thought and adjustment and may cause unresolved emotional conflict within an individual. The ability to adapt to change is required in every stressful situation, positive or negative.

Stress Analysis

Even if you are currently not dealing with depression, you most likely are under a great deal of stress due to fibromyalgia complications. The accompanying "Stress Analysis Questionnaire" (see sidebar) was specifically designed to assist you with your health status evaluation. Please be precise and objective with your answers. They should describe your exact present condition and not as you would prefer to be.

Stress Analysis Questionnaire

Stress Risk Factors:

_ Headaches   _ Neck Pain
_ Shoulder Pain   _ Auto Accident
_ Work Injury   _ Backaches
_ Other

Complete the following questions. If the answer is "maybe," check "yes."

Yes	No	**General Stress**
_	_	1. Are you generally dissatisfied with your job, occupation or relations with the opposite sex?
_	_	2. Do you have trouble relaxing or falling asleep?
_	_	3. Do you have trouble concentrating or remembering things?
_	_	4. Do you feel fatigued late in the day?
_	_	5. Do you have headaches, neck or back pain more than two times monthly?
_	_	6. Do you take pain relievers, antacids, tranquilizers, sinus or any other medicine more than two times monthly?
_	_	7. Do you have insomnia or don't sleep enough?
_	_	8. Do you depend on sugar or caffeine stimulants?
_	_	9. Do you lose your temper or become angry easily?
_	_	10. Have you suffered a significant loss in the last year: job, money, divorce, death of loved one?
_	_	11. Do you eat red meat daily?
_	_	12. Is your weight abnormal?
_	_	13. Are you moody?
_	_	14. Are you hyperactive?
_	_	15. Do your hands or feet ever tingle, ache or burn?
_	_	16. Do you have high blood pressure, heart disease, ulcers, colitis or other stress related diseases?
_	_	17. Is there conflict, upset or disappointment in a close personal relationship?
_	_	18. Does eating lack enjoyment for you?
_	_	19. Do you crave sugar?

_ _ 20. Do you take laxatives?
_ _ 21. Would you call yourself a worrier?
_ _ 22. Do you crave sweets?
_ _ 23. Do you get tired after you eat sweets?
_ _ 24. Do you find it difficult to work under pressure?
_ _ 25. Do you develop bruises for no reason?
_ _ 26. Do you have brown spots on your skin?
_ _ 27. Do you sigh or yawn often?
_ _ 28. Does your skin itch?
_ _ 29. Is your sex drive low?
_ _ 30. Do you suffer from skin rashes?
_ _ 31. Do you smoke?
_ _ 32. Do you suffer from acne?

Immune Stress

_ _ 1. Do you get ear infections often?
_ _ 2. Do you suffer with sinus problems?
_ _ 3. Do you have chronic cough?
_ _ 4. Do you get chest colds often?
_ _ 5. Do you get sore throats often?
_ _ 6. Do cuts or scrapes heal slowly?
_ _ 7. Are you chronically tired?
_ _ 8. Do you have frequent allergies?
_ _ 9. Do you get cold sores frequently?
_ _ 10. Do you or have you had bladder/kidney infections?

Digestive Stress

_ _ 1. Do you have a poor appetite?
_ _ 2. Do you experience digestive problems when eating fatty or greasy foods?
_ _ 3. Do you suffer from nausea?
_ _ 4. Does food feel like it lies on your stomach?
_ _ 5. Do you have bad breath?
_ _ 6. Do you have loose bowel movements?
_ _ 7. Are you troubled by heartburn?
_ _ 8. Are you troubled by belching or gas?
_ _ 9. Do you suffer from constipation?
_ _ 10. Have you lost your taste for food?

Circulatory Stress

1. Do you ever get light-headed or dizzy?
2. Do you get pain or tightness in your chest?
3. Do you have low or high blood pressure?
4. Do you get short of breath easily?
5. Do you take prescription heart medication?
6. Does your heart beat fast for no reason?
7. Are your ankles swollen in the morning?
8. Do you have varicose veins?
9. Do you get dizzy when changing positions?

Endocrine Stress

1. Do you get depressed easily?
2. Do you find it difficult to relax?
3. Do you lose your temper easily?
4. Do you cry easily?
5. Do you find it hard to concentrate?
6. Are you in menopause or suffer with PMS?
7. Do you have pain with your cycle?
8. Do you have "abnormal" menstrual flow?
9. Do you have an irregular menstrual cycle?
10. Do you get tired before you eat?
11. Do you have lumps in your breasts?
12. Do you gain weight easily or find it difficult to gain weight?
13. Do you suffer from headaches?

Analyze your answers, and you may, in fact, discover some stressful areas of which you were unaware, thus assisting you in coping more effectively and enhancing the potential of improving your personal health.

If you answered "yes" to three or more of the questions in any one category, lifestyle changes within that area are probably in order for improvement of your general well-being. The answers you provide in this analysis are important in understanding related health matters.

Program for Personal Stress Management

Since stress is a response to event, not just an event that has occurred, good stress management techniques can help you control stress. So even if you can't control the evens that trigger stress responses, you can mediate those responses and even eliminate them.

Sources of and Suggestions for Dealing with Stress

Recognizing situations that are personally stressful is an important first step. How you choose to deal with each is even more important. The following are areas of life that can be stress producing:

1. *Financial affairs.* Avoid debt, manage finances and use discipline with the help of a realistic budget.

2. *Family life.* Work at healthy relationships, communication skills and the art of giving.

3. *Personal and social lives.* Develop a support system through friends and hobbies. Do not harbor resentment, be forgiving and work at boosting your self-esteem.

4. *Physical problems.* Have medical check-ups regularly. If you are experiencing constant fatigue, check your rest habits, improve your nutrition and take supplements in the form of vitamins, minerals and herbs. Exercise regularly, a minimum of four to five times per week. Seek professional advice in all the above areas.

5. *Work life.* If you are unhappy with your work, investigate continuing education and job training opportunities to improve where you are. If you strongly feel you are misplaced, then courageously seek your purpose and pursue

your new mission with a passion. Consider your work as a joy and pleasure.

6. *Change.* Change is inevitable; therefore, develop a positive attitude toward change. Remember that change can be healthy. Take care to make changes slowly and not too many at once to ensure success.

7. *Time pressures.* Much of our stress is caused by mismanagement of time, procrastination and deadlines. Try to find a schedule that works for you.

Since stress can lead directly to depression, we need to focus on how to overcome stress. One of the keys to successful stress management is to develop the positive habit of awakening each day with a thankful heart and an optimistic attitude. As you first begin to gain consciousness in the early morning, the subconscious mind is functioning at the alpha level, ten to twelve brain wavelengths per second. The subconscious mind then is more sensitive and receptive to thoughts, emotions and aspirations than at any other time. Therefore, it is at this part of the day that you want to visualize yourself pain free, happy, optimistic, productive and successful. These thoughts and aspirations will go with you throughout the day. Also remember that your very thoughts and emotions are triggering the release of endorphins and catecholamines, the healing and uplifting hormones within your immune system. By focusing on all that is hopeful, joyful, pleasant, loving and optimistic, you can take the edge off stress and continuously improve the condition and state of fibromyalgia as you consistently move toward a healthy existence. The list below contains some other guidelines for a healthful stress management program:

- *Boost your nutrition* by eating more frequently, four or more times per day. Eat with balance by choosing an abundance of complex carbohydrates and high fiber foods such as whole grains, whole grain breads and cereals, rice, pasta, beans, peas and potatoes, along with plenty of fresh fruits and vegetables. Be sure only 20 percent of your total daily diet contains fat. Avoid sugar, alcohol, tobacco and caffeine.

• *Take a nutritional supplement.* Vitamin and mineral supplements of any antioxidant combination will boost the immune system and enhance the cellular cleansing process by maintaining and invigorating cellular energy, cardiovascular awareness and youthful vitality.

• *Get regular exercise.* Exercise aerobically by cycling, walking or swimming a minimum of four to five times per week. Also, include stretching and muscle toning exercises two to three days per week. Joint stretching and muscle toning exercises will be very beneficial and remember that exercising regularly will increase the potential for the fibromyalgia victim to move into deep sleep while resting.

• *Balance rest and relaxation* with your exercise and other activities. Be sure to get adequate amounts of sleep, focus on the positive, work at sleeping peacefully by going through your relaxation exercises while visualizing your goals. Remember that rest and relaxation will help to reduce muscle tension, which will help in reducing pain.

• *Avoid prescription tranquilizers and sleeping medications.* While these may help you get to sleep, they will suppress deep sleep and often make fibromyalgia symptoms worse. Alcohol or narcotic pain medications taken in the evenings have the same effect on deep sleep and also should be avoided.

• *Practice good stress management techniques.* Don't over extend yourself, and always plan ahead for difficult tasks. Remember to ask for help whenever needed. Limit your responsibilities and activities to manageable levels.

- *Be especially moderate with caffeine and alcoholic beverages,* and do not use drugs unless prescribed by your doctor.

- *Ingest a reasonable number of calories* to enhance your weight maintenance program.

Stress Reducing Techniques

The art of relaxation is most important in stress management and can be a structured or an informal technique. The following are some proven stress reducing activities:

- gentle stretching
- a brief nap
- ocean or nature sounds
- doing a favor for a friend
- meditation, prayer
- using a foot massager
- a warm bath
- a walk in the woods
- relaxing music
- using humor frequently
- mental relaxation
- breathing/muscle relaxation

The Depression Side Effect

Not surprisingly, fibromyalgia is generally viewed as a negative stressor, as is most anything that threatens disability, produces pain and limits one's ability to function normally. Depression is a common side effect. Many researchers, in fact, believe that when one is threatened with disability or loss of normal function, this is much more likely to induce depression than is the pain from the condition itself.

Depression generally includes a wide variety of emotional disorders ranging from mild to severe. There are three basic levels of severity. First, some individuals become depressed on a one-time only basis. The depression can last for a day, a few days or several weeks, but it never returns. Recurrent depressive disorders, the second type, can appear and disappear peri-

"I carry your book everywhere I go"

Thanks for writing your book, *Reversing Fibromyalgia*. I have searched for these answers for years. This is the only treatment regimen I have found to turn me back toward health and vitality. I have my life back! I carry your book everywhere I go—it has become my fibromyalgia Bible.
Deborah
North Carolina

odically, leaving one feeling very good and normal between the episodes of depression. Finally, chronic depressive disorders can last for several years, maybe even for half a lifetime or more. Very often the symptoms are more severe in the first two to four years.

What doctors call *subclinical depression* is not serious enough to lead to diagnosis or treatment. Clinical depression, however, means that your symptoms are serious enough to warrant medical attention and treatment. Only your physician or psychologist should make that determination. Remember, however, if the number of subclinical symptoms continues to increase, or if they seem to become more severe, then treatment could be warranted in this case as well (O'Koon, 1996).

Recognizing the Symptoms of Depression

If you experience symptoms of depression, and they do not seem to go away or seem to worsen, then you could possibly truly have the condition of clinical depression. The following is a list of the symptoms of depression to look for. If you one or more of these symptoms for an extended period of time, then you should contact your physician right away (Fries, 1995):

- loss of interest in the things you normally enjoy
- lack of interest in sex
- irritability or blue moods
- restlessness or a slowed-down feeling
- feelings of worthlessness or guilt
- appetite changes leading to weight gain or loss
- suicidal thoughts or thoughts of dying
- problems with concentration, thinking or memory
- difficulty making decisions
- lack of sleep or sleeping too much
- constant lack of energy
- headaches not caused by any other disease or condition
- other aches and pains not caused by any other condition
- digestive problems unrelated to any other condition
- feelings of hopelessness
- anxiety
- low self-esteem
- nightmares, especially with themes of loss, pain or death
- preoccupation with failure, illness, etc.
- fear of being alone

Who Is at High Risk for Depression?

Physicians and psychologists have identified specific risk factors that increase the odds of depression (O'Koon 1996). These apply to the general population and not just fibromyalgia sufferers. You have an increased risk for depression if you:

- are a woman.
- have had a prior depressive episode.
- had your first depressive episode before you were forty years old.
- have a medical condition.
- have just given birth.
- have very little or no social support.

- have undergone a stressful life event (positive or negative).
- abuse alcohol or drugs.
- have a family history of depressive disorders.
- received only partial relief from an earlier episode of depression.
- have ever attempted suicide.

The above list of risk factors only helps identify those who are more susceptible to depression. They do not mean that if you have some of those risk factors in your life that you are absolutely doomed to depression. It also does not mean that you are guaranteed a depression-free life if the list does not describe you. If you feel that you could possibly be depressed, get medical help immediately and possibly a referral to a therapist. Since certain drugs can help cause depression, inform your physician of the medications that you are currently or have recently been taking.

Dealing with Depression

As mentioned in Chapter 3, antidepressant are often prescribed for fibromyalgia patients but are not always the best option. Each case of depression is different and is caused by a unique combination of factors. Antidepressants may be necessary, but in many cases, they are not, and may cover up symptoms instead of addressing the true causes, according to Rita Elkins, author of *Solving the Depression Puzzle*. Antidepressants also have a number of side effects that may actually aggravate fibromyalgia symptoms.

For those depressed fibromyalgia sufferers who may be considering antidepressants, consider trying alternative treatment methods before using drugs. In fact, if you adopt my nutrition and supplement plans, you may find that the depression disappears with other fibromyalgia symptoms. Sleeping disorders, hormone imbalances, food allergies and irritable bowel may also trigger depression and should be addressed before starting antidepressants.

Exercise is an excellent depression treatment. Several studies have found that exercise is a valuable therapy for mild to moderate depression. Supplements like St. John's wort, SAMe, 5-HTP and DLPA may also be helpful. If you are interested in learning more about fighting depression naturally, Elkin's *Solving the Depression Puzzle* is an excellent reference.

Nutrition to Beat Stress and Depression

- Avoid skipping meals, especially breakfast.
- Limit your intake of sugar and highly refined foods.
- Limit fat intake to 20 percent of your total calories.
- Increase fiber in the form of fruits, vegetables, breads, cereals and legumes. (Do this gradually so as to avoid bloating.)
- Maintain appropriate weight with a balance of 70 percent carbohydrates, 20 percent fats, and 10 percent protein on a daily basis.
- Modify your intake of red meat, caffeine and alcohol.
- Eliminate NutraSweet. (Use honey or fructose instead.)
- Take supplements, including antioxidants. The minimum suggested amounts daily are 1,000 mg of vitamin C, 800 IU of vitamin E, 25,000 IU of beta carotene, 50 mg of coenzyme Q10 and 100 mg per fifty pounds of body weight of pycnogenol (proanthocyanidins).
- Drink 72 ounces of purified water daily. If you have no choice but to drink tap water, refrigerate it to allow the chlorine and other impurities to dissipate. Water in tea and other drinks does not count toward your daily water requirement.

Rest, Worry and Stress

Rest is as vital as exercise and nutrition for general health

"I am now able to fight this disease face-to-face"

I have been suffering from this debilitating disease for over 15 years. Your book has helped me tremendously to understand this disease. Thank you for your empathy and love for your fellowman, and for providing such helpful information that lends understanding and hope for reversal of this disease. Because of you, your book and your compassion, I am now able to fight this disease face-to-face. And, I will not let it beat me.

Lois
Ontario

and combating stress. Research indicates that adults require between six and eight hours of sleep. You should determine whether you require six, seven or eight hours through experimentation and monitoring your sleep over a prolonged period. When you have adequate sleep and the body is rested, you will wake up naturally without an alarm. Try the following for improved rest:

- Exercise regularly, but not too close to bedtime.
- Avoid eating and ingesting stimulants after 6:00 p.m.
- Keep your bedroom quiet and dark.
- Establish a pre-sleep routine (i.e., reading, meditating, praying, etc.).
- Refrain from taking sleeping pills.
- Organize your concerns and develop action plans with objectivity rather than worry.
- Always plan your day in the afternoon or evening of the day before—not the morning of that day.

Fibromyalgia can produce a host of psychological changes due to anxiety, frustration, pain, depression and stress. The reversing fibromyalgia regimen and approach will assist you in healthfully managing stress and avoiding depression in several ways. By utilizing your total fibromyalgia treatment program of nutrition, exercise and suggested supplements, along with the stress management methods and techniques, you should be able to combat stress and overcome and avoid depression.

Final Thoughts

While compiling research for the second edition of this book, I couldn't help but notice the huge leap in the amount of published research on fibromyalgia compared with what was available when *Reversing Fibromyalgia* was first released in 1997. I am pleased with the increased availability of information on fibromyalgia and with the growing acceptance of the syndrome among medical professionals and research scientists.

I hope that my book and the updates have been valuable to you in your education about fibromyalgia and how to treat it, but your education should not stop here. This is just the beginning. New research is being done every day on the syndrome, and if you are serious about reversing your condition, I urge you to continue learning through further reading and research. I have included the Resource Guide at the end of the book to help you begin.

I also want to emphasize how important it is for you to conduct firsthand research from your own experiences. Each case of fibromyalgia is unique, and it is essential for you to be observant and to write down your own experiences with the disease and treatment options. With the help of your doctor, experiment with different therapy combinations, and be specific when writing down the results. Continue those treatments that are beneficial and throw out elements that aren't helping.

Most of all, be patient. It will take time for you to perfect your personalized treatment plan. Although complete recovery won't happen overnight, you should start feeling improvements within weeks if you are diligent and you don't underestimate the mind-body connection. A change in behavior first requires a change in thought, and the spark of physical health also is ignited in the mind. It is a place to begin.

Positive thinking is essential to your success, and you can begin to think positive right now—this very second. So right now, I ask you to really believe in your power to get well. Take a moment and visualize yourself as a healthy person with the potential for a healthy future. If you were healthy right now, what would you most want to do? What will it take to get you to that point, where you can do what you want the most? Be as specific as possible—and then, begin. I hope that if nothing else, this book has given you courage and optimism and have empowered you to change, to heal, to be happy.

Appendix A

Health Risk Appraisal Patient Profile

1. Name any doctor or health care professional who has treated you in the past and their specialization:

1. _____
2. _____
3. _____

Have you been diagnosed with fibromyalgia? __ Yes   __ No
By whom/where?

2. How long have you had symptoms? _____

What symptoms have you experienced?

_____

_____

_____

_____

3. Indicate the areas in which you have pain:

__ Neck   __ Arms   __ Shoulders   __ Hips
__ Back (Upper)   __ Thighs   __ Back (Lower)   __ Knees/Ankles
__ Other

Describe: _____

_____

_____

_____

_____

4. Intensity of Pain - Rate from 1 to 10

Mild 1   2   3   4   5   6   7   8   9   10   Severe

Comments: _____

_____

_____

5. Frequency of Pain: __ Early Morning __ Periodically During the Day

__ Constantly   __ While Sleeping

Comments: _____

_____

_____

6. Do you awaken in the morning __ Fatigued   __ Stiff   __ Achy

Comments: _____

_____

_____

7. Do you experience disrupted sleep patterns? __ Yes   __ No

Are you awakened easily? __ Yes   __ No   _____ How Often?

Comments: _____

_____

_____

8. Do you have frequent eye prescription changes? __ Yes   __ No

If you do not wear glasses, do you have occasional blurring? __ Yes   __ No

Comments: _____

_____

9. Do you experience irritable bladder syndrome? __ Yes __ No

Comments: _____

_____

_____

10. Are you depressed or have you been in the past? __ Yes __ No

Comments: _____

_____

_____

11. Do you have gastrointestinal disturbances? __ Yes __ No

Indigestion? __ Yes __ No
Diarrhea? __ Yes __ No

Comments: _____

_____

_____

12. Do you have numbing & tingling in the hands? __ Yes __ No

Comments: _____

_____

Do you have numbing & tingling in the feet? __ Yes __ No

Comments: _____

_____

Do you have soft tissue swelling? __ Yes __ No

Comments: _____

_____

13. Do you experience PMS? __ Yes __ No
Painful periods? __ Yes __ No

Comments: _____

_____

_____

14. Do you experience muscular spasms or twitching? __ Yes __ No

Comments: _____

_____

_____

15. List any physical or emotional traumatic experiences including illnesses you have experienced:

__ Accident   __ Death in the family   __ Unstable relationship
__ Divorce   __ Bankruptcy   __ Dislike of job
__ Illness/Virus/Surgery

Comments: _____

_____

16. Are you on medication? Please indicate below those you are taking.

Antidepressants

	Mg
__ Amitryptyline	____
__ Elavil	____
__ Zanax	____
__ Zoloft	____
__ Prozac	____

Sleeping Pills & Tranquilizers

	Mg
__ Valium	____
__ Helicon	____
__ Restoril	____
__ Paxil	____
__ Benzodiazepines	____

Corticosteriods

__ Prednisone	____

Acetaminophen

__ Datril	____

__ Cortisone   ____   __ Tylenol   ____

__ Liquiprin   ____

NSAIDS

__ Advil   ____   __ Indocin   ____

__ Motrin   ____   __ Nuprin   ____

__ Aspirin   ____   __ Ibuprofen   ____

__ Excedrin

Comments: _____

_____

17. Do you exercise? __ Yes __ No

What kind? _____

How often? _____

Comments: _____

_____

18. Describe your eating habits (i.e. types of food, times/day, etc)

_____

_____

_____

_____

Patient Notes:

_____

_____

_____

_____

_____

_____

Appendix B: Day-Planning Log (blank)

Day-Planning Log

Date:

GAME PLAN	ACTUAL RESULTS
Meal #1 Breakfast (time:)	Meal #1 Breakfast (time:)
Meal #2 Morning Snack (time:)	Meal #2 Morning Snack (time:)
Meal #3 Lunch (time:)	Meal #3 Lunch (time:)
Meal #4 Afternoon Snack (time:)	Meal #4 Afternoon Snack (time:)
Meal #5 Dinner (time:)	Meal #5 Dinner (time:)
Meal #6 Evening Snack (time:)	Meal #6 Evening Snack (time:)

TOTAL PORTIONS CARBOHYDRATES: 6
TOTAL PORTIONS PROTEIN: 6
TOTAL CUPS PURE WATER: 12

TOTAL PORTIONS CARBOHYDRATES:
TOTAL PORTIONS PROTEIN:
TOTAL CUPS PURE WATER:

SUPPLEMENTS/MEDICATION

NOTES/DIARY

Appendix B, cont.: Day-Planning Log (sample)

Day-Planning Log

Date: 10/15/01
Day 14

GAME PLAN	ACTUAL RESULTS
Meal #1 Breakfast (time: 8 AM)	**Meal #1 Breakfast** (time: 7:30)
oatmeal (rolled oats) orange juice, 3 cups water	oatmeal and OJ 2 cups water
Meal #2 Morning Snack (time: 10:30)	**Meal #2 Morning Snack** (time: 9:30)
12 oz can of Slimfast w/soy protein	1 apple-cranberry Slimfast
Meal #3 Lunch (time: 12 PM)	**Meal #3 Lunch** (time: 12:15)
turkey sandwich fruit, 2 cups of water	turkey sandwich, angel food cake 2 cups of water
Meal #4 Afternoon Snack (time: 2:30)	**Meal #4 Afternoon Snack** (time: 3:00)
nutritional snack bar 3 cups of water	Slimfast bar 2 cups of water
Meal #5 Dinner (time: 5 PM)	**Meal #5 Dinner** (time: 6:30)
grilled salmon, potatoes green salad, 2 cups of water	grilled salmon, green salad w/ olive oil, 2 cups of water
Meal #6 Evening Snack (time: 7:30)	**Meal #6 Evening Snack** (time: 9:00)
small bowl of strawberries 2 cups of water	strawberries w/ banana 1 cup of water
TOTAL PORTIONS CARBOHYDRATES: 6	**TOTAL PORTIONS CARBOHYDRATES:** 6
TOTAL PORTIONS PROTEIN: 6	**TOTAL PORTIONS PROTEIN:** 5
TOTAL CUPS PURE WATER: 12	**TOTAL CUPS PURE WATER:** 9

SUPPLEMENTS/MEDICATION

rice bran extract – 500 mg

grape seed extract – 50 mg

multivitamin, day formula

ibuprofen – 400 mg/pain

magnesium/malic acid 400 mg/each

prescribed antidepressant

NOTES/DIARY

less pain today—feel better

walked 30 min/ 2x today to help
w/sleep

45 min of Body Advantage exercise
giving more strength and
confidence

20 min meditation, early evening
to relieve stress, read novel 1 hr

ask doctor about possibly stopping
antidepressants

Appendix B, cont.: 3-Day Sample Meal Plans

DAY 1
Breakfast
Easy Egg Tortillas:
Saute 1 clove garlic, 1/4 c. chopped onion, 1/4 c. chopped green pepper in 1 T. olive oil for 2 minutes. Add 6 eggs and salt and pepper. Scramble until eggs are cooked. Divide and wrap into 5 tortilla shells, add picante sauce.
Orange or Strawberries
Morning Snack
Mixed Nuts
Lunch
Tuna Salad Sandwich
Fresh Strawberries,Peaches or Cantaloupe
Afternoon Snack
Nutritional Shake with Soy Protein
Dinner
Steamed Mixed Veggies
Baked Potato with Low-fat Sour Cream and/or Pepper
Oatmeal Drop Cookie:
Preheat oven to 400°F. Combine 2 c. spelt flour, 1 1/4 c. Fruitsource, 1 t. baking powder, 1/2 t. soda, 1 t. cinnamon, 3 c. rolled oats, and 1 c. raisins. Stir 3/4 t. stevia into 1/2 c. milk; and add to the dry ingredients. Mix and drop by the teaspoonful onto baking sheet. Bake 10 to 12 minutes.
Evening Snack
Green Salad with Olive Oil and Vinegar

DAY 2
Breakfast
Bowl of 12-Grain Cereal
Glass of Orange or Grapefruit Juice
Morning Snack
Nutritional Shake or Meal Bar
Lunch
Grilled Chicken Sandwich
Fresh Strawberries, Peaches or Cantaloupe

Appendix B, cont.: 3-Day Sample Meal Plans

Afternoon Snack
Mixed Nuts

Dinner
Grilled Salmon:
Place frozen salmon steaks in aluminum foil on top of hot grill. Mix 3/4 c. melted butter, 1/4 c. lemon juice and 1/4 c. fresh minced cilantro leaves. Baste steaks with mixture and cover grill. Turn steaks after 10 minutes. Continue basting until steaks are tender, approximately 20 to 25 minutes.
Garden Salad or Steamed Asparagus
Oatmeal Cookie

Evening Snack
Raw Veggies like Carrots, Broccoli or Celery

DAY 3

Breakfast
Buttermilk Pancakes:
Mix 2 1/2 c. buttermilk, 2 eggs, 1/2 t. salt, and 1 t. baking soda thorougly. Add 3 c. of spelt flour and beat until smooth. Do not over beat. Spoon onto hot griddle sprayed with Pam and cook until top is full of holes and underside is brown. Turn and brown other side. Top with fresh strawberries or blueberries.

Morning Snack
Nutritional Shake

Lunch
Turkey Sandwich
Apple or Banana

Afternoon Snack
Trail Mix or Mixed Nuts

Dinner
Easy Cod Fillets:
Heat oven to 350°F. Bake 10 pieces of frozen cod in baking dish for 25 minutes. Top with 1 c. fat-free mayonnaise and 1/2 c. crushed low-fat Ritz crackers. Bake an additional 15 minutes or until fish is tender and flaky. Top with lemon.
Steamed Broccoli

Evening Snack
Raw veggies like carrots or cucumbers

Glossary of Terms

Acetaminophen: A pain-relieving and fever-reducing drug used in many over-the-counter drugs.

Acupuncture: An ancient Chinese healing art that involves inserting very thin needles into certain points along the body to relieve pain and promote healing.

Acupressure: Application of pressure over specific muscle sites to relieve pain and muscle spasm.

Acute: Begins quickly and is intense or sharp; sharp or severe.

Aerobic: designating activities involving increased oxygen consumption by the body as a result of aerobic exercise and/or exercises involving the legs, i.e., cycling, swimming, and walking.

Acupressure: Application of pressure over specific muscle sites to relieve pain and muscle spasm.

Anaphylaxis: A rare, severe allergic reaction characterized by difficulty in breathing or swelling, a swollen tongue, dizziness, fainting, hives, puffy eyelids, fast and irregular heartbeat or pulse, and/or a change in face color.

Anemia: A reduction to below normal in the number of red blood cells in the blood. A common symptom of anemia is fatigue.

Ankylosing spondylitis: A type of arthritis that primarily affects the spine and sacroiliac joints. Tendons and ligaments may become inflamed where they attach to the bone. Advanced forms may result in the formation of bony bridges between vertebrae, causing the spine to become rigid.

Antibody: A type of blood protein made by the body in response to a foreign substance (antigen). An antibody binds to an antigen and eliminates it from the body.

Antidepressant: A medication utilized in relief of depression or the blues, tricyclic antidepressants help to relieve night-time muscle spasms in fibromyalgia victims.

Antigen: Any substance the body regards as foreign or potentially dangerous, and that results in the production of an antibody.

Antihistamine: Inhibits or counteracts the action of histamine, a biological chemical produced in immune response. Histamine has a powerful effect, i.e., dilating blood vessels and the stimulation of the secretion of gastric juices. These drugs can also cause drowsiness, a serious problem for people with fibromyalgia who are battling stress and fatigue.

Anti-inflammatory drug: A drug, such as aspirin or ibuprofen, that reduces pain, redness, swelling and heat.

Antinuclear antibody test (ANA): A screening test used for several types of inflammatory conditions, and especially useful in detecting systemic lupus erythematosus. It is positive antinuclear antibodies may also be formed in reaction to certain medications, viral infections, liver diseases, various types of arthritis and even aging.

Apnea (Sleep): The hesitation or stopping of breathing during sleep, caused by obstructions within the nasal airway, sometimes occurring a multiple number of times during the night. This condition is also very closely associated with obesity, although not all obese people have sleep apnea. The brain must arouse the sleeper from deep sleep to relieve the obstruction and restore breathing, therefore, sleep apnea has serious health effects such as with the fibromyalgia sufferer.

Arthrodesis: Fixing a joint through surgery to relieve pain or give support; fusion.

Arthroscope: A flexible viewing tube about the diameter of a pencil, inserted through a small incision into the joint capsule, that provides a view of the inside of a joint.

Arthrosopic surgery: Surgery done on a joint using an arthroscope.

Articular: Refers to a joint. (More broadly, it means "the place of junction between two discrete objects.")

Atrophy: Decrease in size of a normally developed organ or tissue; wasting.

Autoimmune disease: A disease due to the action of the immune system against itself, occurring because the immune cells can't differentiate between the body's own material ("self") and that which is foreign ("non-self"). It is possible that certain body proteins are so altered by viral infections, by combination with a drug or chemical, or by extensive trauma, that they are no longer recognizable by the body as "self" and therefore are rejected as foreign.

Biofeedback: A procedure utilizing equipment to monitor the heart rate, skin temperature, muscle tension, and blood pressure. These body signals are exhibited on a monitor or screen so that one can observe how the body is responding. This process or procedure makes one more aware of a reaction to stress and/or pain and to assist the educational process of learning to control the body's physical and emotional reactions.

Biological: A laboratory-concocted agent, similar to the body's own biochemicals and administered in the same manner as drugs, that alters the body's immune response.

Bone spur: A bony growth around the joints seen in people with osteoarthritis. Joints may appear to be swollen.

Bursa: A small sac surrounding the joint and/or located between a tendon and bone. The bursae provide lubrication and reduce friction for joint movement.

Bursitis: Inflammation of the bursas, small, fluid-filled sacs that cushion and reduce friction where muscles and tendons move over bones or ligaments, such as in the shoulders, hips, knees, and elbows.

Carpal tunnel syndrome: A group of symptoms resulting from compression of the medial nerve in the wrist, with pain and burning or tingling numbness in the fingers and hand, sometimes extending to the elbow.

Cartilage: A smooth, resilient tissue that covers the ends of the bones so they don't' rub against each other.

Chondroitin sulfate: A product available in some health-food stores that contains glycosaminoglycans, major structural components of cartilage and connective tissue. Although this product is popular in Europe, there are no good U.S. studies to show it helps rebuild cartilage.

Chromosome: A structure in the nucleus of every cell containing genetic material that determines the characteristics of the cell.

Chronic: Persisting for a long time.

Chronic Fatigue Syndrome (CFS): A condition manifesting fatigue on a long term basis. The symptoms of CFS and fibromyalgia are almost identical with the only difference being the degree of pain that is characteristic in fibromylagia.

Chronobiology: This is the study of rhythms, cycles, and timing of biological events such as secretion of hormones, ovulation, and temperature fluctuations.

Circadian Rhythms: The daily, weekly, monthly, and seasonal schedules on which biological or living things carry out essential tasks such as eating, eliminating, digesting, and growing. Disruption of these rhythms occurs when, for instance, one travels across time zones. This can have a negative and sometimes profound impact on human performance and mood swings.

Clinical ecologist: An allergist with a special interest in environmental influences on health. More commonly known as an environmental physician.

Colchicine: A drug used in the treatment of gout, usually effective in terminating an attack of gout. Side effects may include gastrointestinal symptoms and low blood pressure.

Collagen vascular disease: An autoimmune disease in which the body's fibrous collagen tissues and the cells lining the inside of blood vessels overgrow, causing organ dysfunction and circulation problems.

Complete blood count (CBC): A diagnostic test that measures blood components, including white blood cells, red blood cells and platelets.

Computerized axial tomographic scan (a CT or CAT scan): A sophisticated x-ray imaging technique that produces thin cross-sectional images of body organs.

Connective tissue: a long-fiber type of body tissue that supports and connects internal organs, forms bones and the walls of blood vessels, attaches muscles to bone, and replaces tissues of other types following injury.

Corticosteroids: Hormones produced by the body and closely related to cortisone. Corticosteroids can be synthetically produced and have powerful anti-inflammatory effects. Prednisone and cortisone are two of the synthetic drugs produced by pharmaceutical companies.

Cortisone (corticosteroid): Potent and effective steroid drug related to the hormone cortisol, produced by the adrenal glands. Steroid drugs quickly reduce swelling and inflammation, bud do have possible serious side effects.

Culture: The propagation of microorganisms or living tissue in a special medium conducive to their growth. Fluid withdrawn from a joint might be cultured to see what microorganisms it contains.

Cyclosporine: A drug used to prevent rejection in organ-transplant patients, used with some success in people with rheumatoid arthritis who haven't responded well to other treatments.

Cyst: An enclosed sac or capsule in the body that contains fluid or a semisolid material. Although harmless, a cyst can become infected.

Deep heat: A treatment that uses tissue-penetrating ultrasound waves to heat up small areas of the body. This is the only heat treatment that can penetrate beyond the surface layers of the skin to a joint.

Degenerative joint disease: Osteoarthritis.

Delta Sleep: The deep, restorative, replenishing sleep required for many of the vital body functions such as antibody productions and restorative immune functioning. Disturbances of delta sleep are characteristic of fibromyalgia. The delta waves are brain waves produced during this very deep restorative sleep.

Depression: A state of mind characterized by feelings of worthlessness, irritability, loss of interest in normal activities, lack of sleep, anxiety, low self-esteem, dejection, sadness, and in some cases can be characterized with a preoccupation with loss, pain, death, or other unpleasant themes.

Discoid lupus: A form of lupus that affects only the skin, causing a rash usually across the face and upper part of the body.

Disease-modifying: Altering, changing or slowing the course of a disease.

DMSO (dimethyl sulfoxide): A solvent, unproven to work, that is sometimes applied to swollen, painful joints.

Echocardiogram: A test that uses sound waves to detect fluid around the heart and other heart abnormalities.

Eicosapentaenoic acid (EPA): Omega-3 fatty acids, found in fish such as mackerel, sardines and salmon, and shown to inhibit inflammation in the body.

Environmental physician: A doctor with a special interest in the impact that environment—air, water, food, toxins—has on the health of an individual. These doctors were formerly called clinical ecologists.

Erythrocyte sedimentation rate (see SED Rate): A test that measures how fast red blood cells cling together, fall and settle to the bottom of a test tube. The more inflammatory proteins found in the blood, the faster these cells clump together and sink.

Fibromylagia: A common clinical syndrome of generalized musculoskelatal pain, stiffness, and chronic aching characterized by reproducible tenderness on palpation of specific anatomical sites, generally referred to as tender points. This systemic condition is considered primary when not associated with systemic cause such as trauma, cancer, thyroid disease and pathologies of rheumatic arthritis or connective tissues. The name fibromyalgia has for the most part replaced the term "fibrositis" which was once used to describe the disorder when there was suspicion that inflammation was a part of the fibromylagia condition.

Fibrous: Composed of or containing fibers. (e.g. Ligaments are rubbery bands of strong fibrous tissue.)

Flare-up: A period of time when symptoms worsen.

Gamma-interferon: A medicinal preparation derived from live cells that is being tried experimentally in the treatment of RA and other rheumatic diseases. A biochemical produced by certain of the body's immune cells, gamma-interferon has a range of effect on the body's immune system.

Gamma-linolenic acid (GLA): A fatty acid—found in high concentrations in black-current oil, evening-primrose oil, and borage oil—thought to have anti-inflammatory actions in the body.

Genetic markers: Specific genes or groups of genes on chromosomes that indicate a particular genetic tendency, including a tendency to develop certain types of diseases.

Glycosaminoglycans: Major structural components of cartilage and connective tissue. Available as chondroitin sulfate.

Gold salts: Gold compounds, given by injection or orally, used in the treatment of rheumatoid arthritis.

Gout: A form of arthritis caused by deposits of uric acid crystals in the joint. Gout usually strikes a single joint, often the big toe and often with sudden, severe pain.

Hematocrit: The volume percentage of red blood cells in whole blood.

Hemoglobin: A protein that transports oxygen in the blood.

Hemorrhage: The escape of blood from a ruptured vessel. Hemorrhage can be external, internal or into the skin or other tissues.

Hydroxy chloroquine: An antimalarial drug (brand name Plaquenil) that is used to treat rheumatoid arthritis.

Hypothalamic-Pituitary-Thyroid Axis: The primary brain-hormonal energy production response axes (i.e., the place where brain function and hormonal function are coordinated in response to the need for energy production).

Ibuprofen: A nonsteroid anti-inflammatory agent.

Immunosuppressive: Inhibiting the immune system in a way that interferes with the formation of antibodies.

Immunotoxin: A monoclonal antibody that contains a toxin. The antibody kills a targeted immune cell and thus represses inflammation.

Infectious arthritis: A type of arthritis caused by an infection somewhere in the body. The infection travels to the joint.

Inflammation: The body's protective response to an injury or infection. The classic signs—heat, redness, swelling and pain—are produced as a result of biochemicals secreted by the body's infection-fighting immune cells as they attempt to wall off and destroy any germs, and to break down and remove damaged tissue.

Joint capsule: A tough, fibrous, fluid-filled tissue that completely surrounds a joint. Synovial cells lining the joint capsule secrete fluid that keeps the joint lubricated.

Juvenile rheumatoid arthritis: Any type of arthritis that develops in children. There are several subtypes.

Ligament: A thick, cordlike fiber that attaches to bones to keep them in correct alignment.

Liver biopsy: A surgical procedure that removes a bit of liver tissue for examination. The tissue is procured using a long, hollow-core needle, which is inserted through the skin into the liver.

Lupus: See systemic lupus erythematosus.

Lyme disease: A type of arthritis caused by bacteria transmitted by a tick that infests a variety of animals, including deer, mice and domestic animals such as dogs.

Lymphoma: Cancer of the lymph glands, which are part of the immune system.

Magnetic resonance imaging (MRI): A noninvasive medical procedure that can produce images of soft tissues that would not be seen on an x-ray.

Mast cell: A type of immune cell, often found on the surface linings of organs, that is involved in allergic reactions.

Metabolism: The body's building up of new body tissues from food sources and breaking down of those food sources to deriveenergy. This building up and breaking down, life sustaining process within the body requires the burning of calories and this metabolic rate determines the number of calories burned per hour.

Methotrexate: A powerful drug, with many potential side effects, used in the treatment of rheumatoid arthritis.

Minocycline: A form of the antibiotic tetracycline currently being tested in a clinical trial as a treatment for rheumatoid arthritis.

Monoclonal antibody: A laboratory-replicated antibody being used experimentally to diminish inflammatory reactions in the body.

Myofascial Pain Syndrome: This syndrome describes a localized aria of muscle and surrounding tissue pain and/or tenderness.

Neuritis: Inflammation of nerves.

Nightshade: A botanical family that includes potatoes, eggplants, tomatoes, peppers (red and green bell peppers, chili peppers and paprika). Some people believe the nightshade family can cause joint inflammation.

Nitrates: Food preservatives found in cured meats and some other foods that may cause joint swelling in some people.

Nonsteroidal anti-inflammatory drugs (NSAIDs): A group of drugs having pain-reliving, fever-reducing and anti-inflammatory effects due to their ability to inhibit the synthesis of prostaglandins. Includes aspirin, ibuprofen and many prescription drugs.

Nutritionist: A person who provides nutritional counseling. Although some nutritionists are well trained and knowledgeable, anyone, regardless of training, can call himself a nutritionist.

Occupational therapist: A health-care professional who provides services designed to restore self-care, work and leisure skills of people who have specific performance incapacities.

Omega-3 fatty acids (also called eicosapentaenoic acid, or EPA): Fatty acids found in fish such as mackerel, sardines and salmon, and shown to inhibit inflammation in the body.

Orthopedist (or orthopedic surgeon): A doctor who specializes in surgery of the joints and related structures.

Oscilloscope: An instrument that displays a visual representation of electrical variations on a fluorescent screen.

Osteoarthritis: Degenerative arthritis, often caused by joint injuries or old age. The most common type of arthritis.

Osteonecrosis: Death of bone cells.

Penicillamine: A drug, related to penicillin, that is sometimes used to treat rheumatoid arthritis.

Pericarditis: Inflammation of the pericardium, the fibrous tissue surrounding the heart.

Placebo: A supposedly inert substance, such as a sugar pill or injection of sterile water, that may be given under the guise of effective treatment. In "controlled" clinical research studies, a group of people taking a placebo is compared with a group receiving the treatment being studied. The placebo group is called the "control group." Studies show that about one-third of the people taking a placebo—for any reason—show an improvement in symptoms, at least initially. That phenomenon Is called the "placebo response."

Plaquenil: Brand name for an anti-malaria drug (hydroxy-chloroquine) that is used to treat rheumatoid arthritis.

Platelet: Disk-shaped blood element that tends to adhere to damaged or uneven surfaces and help blood to clot.

Primary-care physician: The doctor you're most likely to see first for most illnesses. May be a general practitioner, a family practitioner or an internist.

Prostaglandin: Hormonelike substance produced in the body from fatty acids. Prostaglandins have a variety of effects, including the control of inflammation.

Psychologist: A nonmedical professional (usually with a Ph.D. in psychology) who may offer various forms of psychotherapy. A psychologist cannot prescribe drugs.

Psychoneuroimmuinology (PNI): A new field of study that is concerned with the mind and how it can affect our immune system's complex network of vessels, internal organs, and white blood cells. The fascinating fact about this field indicates that the vital body systems, the brain and the immune system, communicate through a rich network of blood vessels and influence one another. This field has been created recently by scientists al over the world such as psychiatrists, endocrinologists, neuroscientists, immunologists, and microbiologists that have united their fields of expertise.

Purine: Protein compound, found in anchovies, organ meats, mushrooms and other foods, that can aggravate gout by elevating body levels of uric acid, which crystallizes in joints.

Range-of-motion exercise: Exercise specifically designed to keep a joint flexible.

Registered Dietitian (R.D.): A nutritional counselor who has been certified in dietetics by the American Dietetic Association (ADA).

Remission: Diminution or abatement of the symptoms of a disease.

Revision: An operation to repair or replace an artificial joint that has loosened, broken or become infected.

Rheumatic disease: A condition that involves inflammation and degeneration of connective tissues and related structures. Such diseases can affect the joints, muscles, tendons and ligaments, heart and lungs, skin and eyes, as well as the protective coverings of some internal organs.

Rheumatoid arthritis: A chronic disease with inflammatory changes occurring throughout the body's connective tissues.

Rheumatoid factor: A protein, found in the blood of many people with rheumatoid arthritis, that indicates the presence of inflammation in the body.

Rheumatoid nodule: Small round or oval bump just under the skin found in some people with rheumatoid arthritis.

Rheumatologist: A doctor who specializes in the treatment of arthritis, especially rheumatoid arthritis and other inflammatory diseases.

Sacroiliac joint: The tailbone; five fused vertebrae wedged between the bones of the pelvis.

Scleroderma: A condition that involves thickening of the skin and changes in blood vessels and the immune system.

Solanine: A chemical substance found in plants such as tomatoes and potatoes. In large amounts, solanine may produce joint inflammation.

Splint: A rigid or flexible appliance to immobilize or protect inflamed joints.

Sternum: A plate of bones forming the breastbone.

Steroid drug: Potent drug related to the hormone cortisol, produced by the adrenal glands. Steroid drugs quickly reduce swelling and inflammation, but have possibly serious side effects.

Subchondral bone: Bone found directly under the cartilage of a joint.

Sulfasalazine: A powerful drug used in the treatment of rheumatoid arthritis. In a preliminary study by Dutch researchers, sulfasalazine was found to slow joint destruction in people with early RA.

Symmetrical: Equal in size or shape (of the body or parts of the body); very similar in placement about an axis.

Synovectomy: The cutting out of a synovial membrane of a joint.

Synovial fluid: Fluid secreted by the synovium, the cells lining a joint capsule, which lubricates the joint and helps nourish the cartilage.

Synovial membrane: The cells lining the inside of the joint capsule, which secrete lubricating fluid. In rheumatoid arthritis, the synovial membrane overgrow the joint capsule, invades the cartilage, and begins to secrete biochemicals that can destroy a joint.

Synovium: The synovial membrane. The cells lining the inside of the joint capsule, which secrete lubricating fluid.

Systemic lupus erythematosus (SLE): A chronic, body-wide inflammatory condition that affects the joints, skin, blood, lungs, cardiovascular and nervous systems, and kidneys.

Tendon: A strong band of tissue that connects muscle to bone.

Tendinitis: Inflammation of a tendon.

Transducer: A device that translates one physical quantity, such as pressure or temperature, to an electrical signal.

Triptergium wilfordii (thundervine root): A Chinese herbal remedy for rheumatoid arthritis currently undergoing clinical trials in China.

Ultrasound: A technique in which deep structures of the body are visualized by recording the reflections (echoes) of ultrasonic waves directed into the tissues.

Uric acid crystal: Tiny, needle-shaped particle that forms in a joint when concentrations of uric acid become high, as in gout.

Vasculitis: Inflammation of blood vessels.

Vegan diet: A vegetarian diet that excludes dairy products and eggs.

Visualization: A method of process of thought utilizing the subconscious mind and the imagination to assist in goal achievement, whether it involves family, career, finances, or simply altering positive thinking on a daily basis to enhance the return to health and vitality in one's pursuit of getting well.

Bibliography

Aaron, L.A and D. Buckwald. "A review of the evidence for overlap among unexplained clinical conditions." *Annals Intern Med.* 134, no. 9 part 2 (May 1, 2001): 868–881.

"Absorption and utilization of amino acids." Mendel Friedman, ed. *U.S. Department of Agriculture.* (Albany, NY) vol. I, II, III. Boca Raton, Florida: CRC Press, 1989.

Ackenheil, M. "Genetics and pathophysiology of affective disorders: relationship to fibromyalgia." *Z Rheumatol.* 57, suppl 2 (1998): 5–7.

Alexander, J. W. et al. "Beneficial effects of aggressive protein feeding in severely burned children." *Annals of Surgery.* 192 (1980): 505.

Alfano, A.P. et al. "Static magnetic fields for treatment of fibromyalgia: a randomized controlled trial." *J Altern Complement Med.* 7, no. 1 (February 2001): 53–64.

Anderberg, U.M. and K. Uvnas-Moberg. "Plasma oxytocin levels in female fibromyalgia syndrome patients." *Zeitschrift fur Rheumatologie.* 59, no. 6 (December 2000): 373–379.

Balch, J. F. and P.A. Balch. *Prescription for Nutritional Healing.* New York: Avery Publishing Group, 1990.

Baldessarini, R. J. "Drugs and treatment of psychiatric disorders." *The Pharmacologic Basis of Therapeutics.* L. S. Goodman and A. Gilman, eds. 7th ed. New York: MacMillan, 1985.

Bengtsson, A. and M. Bengtsson. "Regional sympathetic blockade in primary fibromyalgia." *Pain.* 33 (1988): 161.

Bennett, R. M. "Beyond fibromyalgia: ideas on etiology and treatment." *Journal of Rheumatology.* 16, supple 19 (1989): 185.

Bennett, R. M. et al. "Low levels of somatomedin C in patients with the fibromyalgia syndrome: a possible link between sleep and muscle pain." *Arthritis Rheumatology.* 35 (1992): 1113.

Berman, B. M. and J. P. Swyers. "Complementary medicine treatments for fibromyalgia syndrome." *Baillieres Best Pract Res CLin Rheumatol.* 13, no. 3 (1999): 487–492.

Berwaerts, J. et al. "Secretion of growth hormone in patients with chronic fatigue syndrome." *Growth Horm IGF Res.* 8, suppl B (april 1998): 127–129.

Boland, E. W. "Psychogenic rheumatism: the musculoskeletal expression of psychoneurosis." *Annual of Rheumatological Disorders.* 6 (1947): 195.

Bradley, L. A. et al. "Pain complaints in patients with fibromyalgia versus chronic fatigue syndrome." *Curr Rev Pain.* 4, no. 2 (2000): 148–157.

Brand-Miller, Jennie, Ph.D. et al. *The Glucose Revolution.* New York: Marlowe & Company, 1999.

Brooks, P. M. and R.O. Day. "Nonsteroidal anti-inflammatory drugs—differences and similarities." *The New England Journal of Medicine.* 324, no. 24 (June 1991): 1716–1725.

Bucci, L. R. "Reversal of osteoarthritis by nutritional intervention." *ACA Journal of Chiropractic.* 27 (November 1990): 69–72.

Bucci, L. R. *Nutrition Applied to Injury Rehabilitation and Sports Medicine.* Boca Raton, Florida: CRC Press, 1994. pp. 140–149.

Buchwald, D. et al. "The chronic, active epstein-barr virus infection syndrome and primary fibromyal-gia." *Arthritis Rheumatology.* 30 (1987): 1132.

Buckelew, S.P. et al. "Biofeedback/relaxation training and exercise interventions for fibromyalgia: a prospective trial." *Arthritis Care Res.* 11, no. 3 (June 1998): 196–209.

Buskila, D. "Fibromyalgia, chronic fatigue syndrome, and myofascial pain syndrome." *Curr Opin Rheumatol.* 13, no. 2 (March 2001): 117–127.

Calabro, J. J. *Osteoarthritis Diagnosis and Management.* Ch. 18. "Principals of drug therapy." Philadelphia: W. B. Saunders Co., 1992. pp. 317–322

Campbell, S. M. et al. "Clinical characteristics of fibrositis. I. A 'blinded' controlled study of symptoms and tender points." *Arthritis Rheumatology.* 26 (1983): 817.

Carper, J. *Stop Aging Now.* 1st ed. New York: Harper Collins Publishers, 1995.

Chase, T. N. and D. L. Murphy. "Serotonin and central nervous system function." *Annual Review of Pharmacology.* 13 (1973): 181.

Childers, N. F. *Arthritis—A Diet to Stop It: The Nightshades, Aging and Ill Health.* Gainesville, Florida: Horticultural Publications, 1986.

Clark, S.R. et al. "Exercise for patients with fibromyalgia: risks versus benefits." *Curr Rheumatol Rep.* 3, no. 2 (April 2001): 135–140.

Clement, C. D., ed. *Anatomy of the Human Body.* 30th ed. Philadelphia: Lea and Febiger, 1985.

Cousins, Norman. *Anatomy of an Illness: As Perceived by the Patient.* New York: W. W. Norton & Co., 1979.

Cousins, Norman. *The Healing Heart.* New York: W.W. Norton & Co., 1983.

Crofford, L. J. and B. E. Appleton. "Complementary and alternative therapies for fibromyalgia." *Current Rheumatology Reports.* 3, no. 2 (April 2001): 147–156.

Crofford, L. J. et al. "Hypothalamic-pituitary-adrenal axis perturbations in patients with fibromyalgia." *Arthritis Rheumatology.* 37 (1994): 1583–1592.

Dessein, P. H. et al. "Hyposecretion of adrenal androgens and the relation of serum adrenal steroids, serotonin and insulin-like growth factor-1 to clinical features in women with fibromyalgia." *Pain.* 83, no. 2 (November 1999): 313–319.

De Stefano, R. et al. "Image analysis quantification of substance P immunoreactivity in the trapezius muscle of patients with fibromyalgia and myofascial pain syndrome." *J Rheumatol.* 27, no. 12 (December 2000): 2906–2910.

Dexter, P. and K. Brandt. "Distribution and predictors of depressive symptoms of osteoarthritis." *Journal of Rheumatology.* 21, no. 2 (1994): 279–286.

Dollwet, H. H. A. *The Copper Bracelet and Arthritis.* New York: Vantage Press, 1981.

Dunne, F. J. and C. A. Dunne "Fibromyalgia syndrome and psychiatric disorder." *British Journal of Hospital Medicine.* 54 (1995): 194–197.

Elkins, Rita, M.H. *Solving the Depression Puzzle.* Pleasant Grove, Utah: Woodland Publishing, 2001.

Elrod, J. M. *The Body Advantage: Total Wellness System.* Montgomery, Alabama: Dr. Joe M. Elrod and Associates, 1996.

Elrod, J. M. "How not to be a dropout." Newsletter. *Sportrooms of America.* 3 (1982): 27.

Ernberg, M. et al. "Plasma and serum serotonin levels and their relationship to orofacial pain and anxiety in fibromyalgia." *J Orofac Pain.* 14, no. 1 (Winter 2000): 37–46.

Evengard, B. et al. "Chronic fatigue syndrome differs from fibromyalgia. No evidence for elevated substance P levels in cerebrospinal fluid of patients with chronic fatigue syndrome." *Pain.* 78, no. 2 (November 1998): 153–155.

Ferraccioli, G. F. et al. "EMG biofeedback in fibromyalgia syndrome." *Journal of Rheumatology.* 16 (1989): 1013.

Fischbach, F. A. *Manual of Laboratory Diagnostic Tests.* 3rd ed. Philadelphia: J. B. Lippincott, 1991.

Friedberg, F. and L. A. Jason. "Chronic fatigue syndrome and fibromyalgia: clinical assessment and treatment." *J Clin Psychol.* 57, no. 4 (April 2001): 433–455.

Gans, D. A. "Sucrose and delinquent behavior: coincidence or consequence?" *Critical Reviews in Food Science and Nutrition.* 30, no. 1 (1991): 23–48.

Garnett, L. R. "Strong medicine." *Harvard Health Letter.* 1995: 4–6.

Gay, G. "Another side effect of NSAIDs." *Journal of the American Medical Association.* 264, no. 20 (November 28, 1990): 2677–2678.

Germaine, B. F., M.D. "Silicone breast implants and rheumatic disease." *Bulletin on the Rheumatic Diseases.* 41(October 1991): 1–4.

Gold, P. W., M.D. "Stress response and the regulation of inflammatory disease." *Annals of Internal Medicine.* 117 (November 15, 1992): 854–66.

Gowers, W. R. "Lumbago—its lessons and analogues." *British Medical Journal.* 1 (1904): 117.

Goldenberg, D. L. et al. "A randomized controlled trial of amitriptyline and naproxen in the treatment of patients with fibromyalgia." *Arthritis Rheumatology.* 29 (1986): 1371.

Goldenberg, D. L. "Psychological symptoms and psychiatric diagnosis in patients with fibromyalgia." *Journal of Rheumatology.* 16, suppl 19 (1989): 127.

Goldenberg, D. L. "Fibromyalgia and chronic fatigue syndrome: are they the same?" *Journal of Musculoskeletal Medicine.* 7 (1990): 19.

Goldenberg, D. L. et al. "High frequency of fibromyalgia in patients with chronic fatigue seen in a primary care practice." *Arthritis Rheumatology.* 33 (1990): 1132.

Goldenberg, D. L. et al. "The impact of cognitive-behavioral therapy on fibromyalgia." *Arthritis Rheumatology.* 34, suppl 9 (1991): S190.

Goldenberg, D. L. "Fibromyalgia: treatment programs." *Journal of Musculoskeletal Pain.* 1, no. 3/4 (1993): 71.

Goldenberg, D. et al. "A randomized, double-blind crossover trial of fluoxetine and amitriptyline in the treatment of fibromyalgia." *Arthritis Rheumatology.* 39 (1996): 1852.

Granges, G. and G. Littlejohn. "Prevalence of myofascial pain syndrome in fibromyalgia syndrome and regional pain syndrome: a comparative study." *Journal of Musculoskeletal Pain.* 1, no. 2 (1993): 19.

Hadhazy, V. A. et al. "Mind-body therapies for the treatment of fibromyalgia. A systematic review." *J Rheumatol.* 27, no. 12 (2000): 2911–2918.

Hakkinen, A. et al. "Strength training induced adaptations in neuromuscular function of premenopausal women with fibromyalgia: comparison with health women." *Ann Rheum Dis.* 60, no. 1 (January 2001): 21–26.

Hammerly, Milton, M.D. *Fibromyalgia: How to Combine the Best of Traditional and Alternative Therapies.* Holbrook, Massachusetts: Adams Media Corporation, 2000.

Harrison S. and P. Geppetti. "Substance p." *Int J Biochem Cell Biol.* 33, no. 6 (June 2001): 555–576.

Hauri, P. and D. R. Hawkins. "Alpha-delta sleep." *Electroenceph Clin Neurophysiology.* 34 (1973): 233.

Heim, C. et al. "The potential role of hypocortisolism in the pathophysiology of stress-related bodily disorders." *Psychoneuroendocrinology.* 25, no 1 (January 2000): 1–35.

Hendler, N. and A. L. Kolodny. "Using medication wisely in chronic pain." *Patient Care.* 6 (May 1992): 125–139.

Hendler, S. S., M.D. *The Doctor's Vitamin and Mineral Encyclopedia.* New York: Simon and Schuster, 1990.

Hess, E. V., M.D., and A. Mongey, M.D. "Drug-related lupus." *Bulletin on the Rheumatic Diseases.* 40(August 1991): 1–7.

Hobson, J. A. "Sleep after exercise." *Science.* 162 (1968): 1503.

Hodgkinson, R. and D. Woolf. "A five year clinical trial of indomethacin in osteoarthritis of the hip joint." *ACTA Orhtop Scand.* [AU: PLS. Confirm] 50 (1979): 169.

Jaeschke, R. et al. "Clinical usefulness of amitriptyline in fibromyalgia: the results of 23 N-of-1 randomized, controlled trials." *Journal of Rheumatology.* 18 (1991): 447–451.

Jentoft, E. S. et al. "Effects of pool-based and land-based aerobic exercise on women with fibromyalgia/chronic widespread muscle pain." *Arthritis Rheum.* 45, no. 1 (February 2001): 42–47.

Katz, R. S. and H. M. Kravitz. "Fibromyalgia, depression, and alcoholism: a family history study." *J Rheumatol.* 23, no. 1 (January 1996): 149–154.

Kelley, W., M.D., et al. *Textbook of Rheumatology.* Philadelphia: W. B. Saunders, 1989.

Landis, C. A. et al. "Decreased nocturnal levels of prolactin and growth hormone in women with fibromyalgia." *J Clin Endocrinol Metab.* 86, no. 4 (April 2001): 1672–1678.

Legangneux, E. et al. "Cerebrospinal fluid biogenic amine metabolites, plasma-rich platelet serotonin and." *Rheumatology.* 40, no. 3 (March 2001): 290–296.

Lehninger, A. L. Biochemistry. *The John Hopkins University School of Medicine.* 6th ed. New York: Worth Publishers, Inc., 1972.

Littlejohn, G. "Fibromyalgia. What is it and how do we treat it?" *Aust Fam Physician.* 30, no. 4 (April 2001): 327–333.

Mankin, H. J. *Arthritis Surgery: Clinical Features of Osteoarthritis.* Philadelphia: W. B. Saunders Co., 1994. pp. 469–479.

May, K. P. et al. "Sleep apnea in male patients with the fibromyalgia syndrome." *American Journal of Medicine.* 94 (1993): 505.

McBeth, J. and A. J. Silman. "The role of psychiatric disorders in fibromyalgia." *Curr Rheumatol Rep.* 3, no. 2 (April 2001): 157–164.

McCain, G. A. et al. "A controlled study of the effects of a supervised cardiovascular fitness training program on manifestations of primary fibromyalgia." *Arthritis Rheumatology.* 31 (1988): 1135.

McCarty, D. J., M.D. *Arthritis and Allied Conditions: A Textbook of Rheumatology.* 11th ed. Philadelpha: Lea and Febiger, 1989.

Meyer, Scott. "The stress syndrome: research proving stress can sicken you in variety of ways." *Health Scout.* Monday, July 29, 2001. http://www.healthscout.com.

Miller, B., M.D., and C. B. Keane, R.N. *Encyclopedia and Dictionary of Medicine, Nursing and Allied Health.* 4th ed. Philadelphia: W. B. Saunders, 1987.

Moldofsky, H. D. et al. "Musculoskeletal symptoms and non-REM sleep disturbance in patients with 'fibrositis syndrome' and healthy subjects." *Psychosomatic Medicine.* 37 (1975): 341.

Moldofsky, H. D. "A chronobiologic theory of fibromyalgia." *Journal of Musculoskeletal Pain.* 1, no. 3/4 (1993): 49.

Moldofsky, H. D. "Sleep, neuroimmune and neuroendocrine functions in fibromyalgia and chronic fatigue syndrome." *Advances in Neuroimmunology.* 5 (1995): 39–56.

Mozes, Alan. "Antidepressants may help fibromyalgia patients." *Reuters Health.* March 19, 2001.

Mozes, Alan. "Meditation may help fibromyalgia patients." *Reuters Health.* March 14, 2001.

Mueller, H. H. et al. "Treatment of fibromyalgia incorporating EEG-Driven stimulation: a clinical outcomes study." *J Clin Psychol.* 57, no. 7 (July 2001): 933–952.

Mur, E. et al. "Electromyography biofeedback therapy in fibromyalgia." *Wien Med Wochenschr.* 149, no. 19–20 (1999): 561–563.

Naschitz, J. E. et al. "Cardiovascular response to upright tilt in fibromyalgia differs from that in chronic fatigue syndrome." *J Rheumatol.* 28, no. 6 (June 2001): 1356–1360.

Nasralla, M. et al. "Multiple mycoplasmal infections detected in blood of patients with chronic fatigue syndrome and/or fibromyalgia syndrome." *Eur J Clin Microbiol Infect Dis.* 18, no. 12 (December 1999): 859–865.

National Research Council. Recommended Dietary Allowances. Academy of Sciences: Washington, DC, 1980. p. 1.

Neumann, L. et al. "The effect of balneotherapy at the Dead Sea on the quality of life of patients with fibromyalgia symptoms." *Clin Rheumatol.* 20, no. 1 (2001): 15–19.

Nilsson, E. et al. "Blood dehydroepiandrosterone sulphate (DHEAS) levels in polymyalgia rheumatica/giant cell arteritis and primary fibromyalgia." *Clin Exp Rheumatol.* 12, no. 4 (July–August 1994): 415–417.

Novak, K. K. et al. *Drug Facts and Comparisons.* St. Louis, MO: Facts and Comparisons, Inc., 1995.

Norregaard, J. et al. "A randomized controlled trial of citalopram in the treatment of fibromyalgia." *Pain.* 61 (1995): 445–9.

Offenbacher, M. and G. Stucki. "Physical therapy in the treatment of fibromyalgia." *Scand J Rheumatol Suppl.* 113 (2000): 78–85.

Offenbaecher, M. et al. "Possible association of fibromyalgia with a polymorphism in the serotonin transporter gene regulatory region." *Arthritis Rheum.* 42, no. 11 (November 1999): 2482–2488.

Offenbaecher, M. et al. "Self-reported depression, familial history of depression and fibromyalgia (FM), and psychological distress in patients with FM." *Z Rheumatol.* 57, suppl 2 (1998): 94–96.

Olson, G. B. et al. "The effects of collagen hydrolysat on symptoms of chronic fibromyalgia and temporomandibular joint pain." *Cranio.* 18, no. 2 (April 2000): 135–141.

O'Malley, P. G. "Treatment of fibromyalgia with antidepressants: a meta-analysis." *J Gen Intern Med.* 15, no. 9 (September 2000): 659–666.

Palm, O. et al. "Fibromyalgia and chronic widespread pain in patients with inflammatory bowel disease: a cross sectional population survey." *J Rheumatol.* 28, no. 3 (March 2001): 590–594.

Panush, R. S., M.D., ed. *Rheumatic Disease Clinics of North America: Nutrition and Rheumatic Diseases.* Philadelphia: W. B. Saunders, 17(May 1991).

Panush, R. S., M.D. "Food-induced ('allergic') arthritis: inflammatory arthritis exacerbated by milk." *Arthritis and Rheumatism.* (February 1986): 220–6.

Panush, R. S., M.D. "Food-induced ('allergic') arthritis: clinical and serologic studies." *Journal of Rheumatology.* 17, no. 3 (1990): 291–4.

Park, J.H. et al. "Evidence for metabolic abnormalities in the muscles of patients with fibromyalgia." *Curr Rheumatol Rep.* 2, no. 2 (April 2000): 131–140.

Pellegrino, M. J. et al. "Familial occurrence of primary fibromyalgia." *Arch Phys Med Rehabilitation.* 70 (1989): 61.

Pellegrino, Mark J., M.D. *Inside Fibromyalgia.* Columbus, Ohio: Anadem Publishing, 2001.

Pisetsky, D., M.D. *The Duke University Medical Center Book of Arthritis.* New York: Fawcett Columbine, 1991.

Quillin, P. "The role of nutrition in cancer treatment." *Health Councilor.* 4(6).

Quillin, P. *Healing Nutrients.* Chicago, Illinois: Contemporary Books, Inc., 1987.

Reeves, K. D. and K. Hassanein. "Randomized prospective double-blind placebo-controlled study of dextrose prolotherapy for knee osteoarthritis with or without ACL laxity." *Altern Ther Health Med.* 6, no. 2 (March 2000): 68–74, 77–80.

Remington, Julianne. "New research on fibromyalgia." January 31, 2001. http://www.americasdoctor.com.

Rooney, T. and P. Rooney. *The Arthritis Handbook.* New York: Balantine Books, 1986.

Russell, I. J. et al. "Treatment of primary fibrositis/ fibromyalgia syndrome with ibuprofen and alprazolam—a double-blind, placebo-controlled study." *Arthritis Rheumatology.* 34 (1991): 552.

Russell, I. J. et al. "Elevated cerebrospinal fluid levels of substance P in patients with the fibromyalgia syndrome." *Arthritis Rheumatology.* 37 (1994): 1593–1601.

Russell, I. J. "Neurochemical pathogenesis of fibromyalgia syndrome." *Journal of Musculoskeletal Pain.* 4 (1996): 61–92.

Sandler, D. P. "Analgesic use and chronic renal disease." *The New England Journal of Medicine.* 320 (1989): 1238–1243.

Saskin, P. et al. "Sleep and post-traumatic rheumatic pain modulation disorder (fibrositis syndrome)." *Psychosomatic Medicine.* 48 (1986): 319.

Schroder, H. D. et al. "Muscle biopsy in fibromyalgia." *Journal of Musculoskeletal Pain.* 1, no. 3/4 (1993): 165.

Schumacher, H. R., M.D., ed. *Primer on the Rheumatic Diseases.* 9th ed. Atlanta: The Arthritis Foundation, 1988.

Sciarillo, W. G. "Lead exposure and child behavior." *American Journal of Public Health.* 82, no. 10 (1992): 1356–1359.

Sheon, R. P., M.D. et al. *Coping With Arthritis.* New York: McGraw-Hill, 1987.

Simms, R. W. et al. "Lack of association between fibromyalgia syndrome and abnormalities in muscle energy metabolism." *Arthritis Rheumatology.* 37 (1994): 801–807.

Simonton, O. et al. *Getting Well Again.* 3rd ed. New York: Bantam Books, 1992.

Simonton, O. and S. Simonton. "Belief systems and management of the emotional aspects of malignancy." *Journal of Transpersonal Psychology.* 7, no. 1 (1975): 29–47.

Smythe, H. "Fibrositis syndrome: a historical perspective." *Journal of Rheumatology.* 16, supple 19 (1989): 2.

Sobel, D. and A. C. Klein. *Arthritis: What Works.* New York: St. Martin's Press, 1989.

St. Amand, R. Paul, M.D. *What Your Doctor May Not Tell You About Fibromyalgia.* New York: Warner Books, 1999.

Stehlin, D. "How to take your medicine—nonsteroidal anti-inflammatory drugs." *FDA Consumer.* June 1990. pp. 33–34.

Stinnett, J. D. *Proteins and Amino Acids-Prospects for Nutritional Therapy in Infection, In Relevance of Nutrition to Sepis.* J. E. Fischer, ed. Columbia, Ohio: Ross Laboratories, 1982.

Tenney, L. *The Encyclopedia of Natural Remedies.* Pleasant Grove, Utah: Woodland Publishing Co, 1995.

"The 5-a-day easy eating plan." *The Johns Hopkins Medical Letter.,* 5, no. 2 (April 1993).

U.S. Department of Health, Education, and Welfare. *Healthy People. 101.* U.S. Government Printing Office, 79-55071, Washington, DC, 1979.

Theodosakis, J., B. Adderly and B. Fox. *The Arthritis Cure.* Ch. 5. "The problem with pain killers." New York: St. Martin's Press, 1997. pp. 69–80.

Torpy, D. J. et al. "Responses of the sympathetic nervous system and the hypothalamic-pituitary-adrenal axis to interleukin-6: a pilot study in fibromyalgia." *Arthritis Rheum.* 43, no. 4 (April 2000): 872–880.

Van Houdenhove, B. et al. "Victimization in chronic fatigue syndrome and fibromyalgia in tertiary care: a controlled study on prevalence and characteristics." *Psychosomatics*. 42, no. 1 (January-February 2001): 21–28.

Vestergaard-Poulsen, P. et al. "31P NMR spectroscopy and electromyography during exercise and recovery in patients with fibromyalgia." *Journal of Rheumatology*. 22 (1995): 1544–1551.

Wallace, D. J. et al. "Cytokines play an aetiopathogenetic role in fibromyalgia: a hypothesis and pilot study." *Rheumatology*. 40, no. 7 (July 2001): 743–749.

Wallace, D. J. et al. "Fibromyalgia, cytokines, fatigue syndromes, and immune regulation." *Advances in Pain Research and Therapy*. J. R. Fricton and E. Awad, eds. Vol. 17. Raven Press, 1990. 227–287.

Weil, A., M.D. *Natural Health, Natural Medicine*. Boston: Houghton Mifflin, 1990.

Weintraub, S., N.D. *Natural Treatments for ADD and Hyperactivity*. Pleasant Grove, Utah: Woodland Publishing, 1997.

Werbach, M. *Nutritional Influences on Illness*. Tarzana, California: Third Line Press, 1988.

Werle, E. et al. "Antibodies against serotonin have no diagnostic relevance in patients with fibromyalgia syndrome." *J Rheumatol*. 28, no. 3 (March 2001): 595–600.

White, K. P. and M. Harth. "Classification, epidemiology, and natural history of fibromyalgia." *Curr Pain Headache Rep*. 5, no. 4 (August 2001): 320–329.

White, K. P. et al. "Work disability evaluation and the fibromyalgia syndrome." *Semin Arthritis Rheumatology*. 24 (1995): 371–381.

Wittrup, I. H. et al. "Comparison of viral antibodies in 2 groups of patients with fibromyalgia." *J Rheumatol*. 28, no. 3 (March 2001): 601–603.

Wolfe, F. "Fibromyalgia: the clinical syndrome." *Rheumatology Dis Clin North America*. 15 (1989): 1.

Wolfe F. et al. "The American College of Rheumatology 1990 criteria for the classification of fibromyalgia: report of the multicenter criteria committee." *Arthritis Rheumatology*. 33 (1990): 160–172.

Wolfe, F. "Fibromyalgia: on diagnosis and certainty." *Journal of Musculoskeletal Pain*. 1, no. 3/4 (1993): 17.

Wolfe, F. "The epidemiology of fibromyalgia." *Journal of Musculoskeletal Pain*. 1, no. 3/4 (1993): 137.

Wolfe, F. et al. "A double-blind placebo controlled trial of fluoxetine in fibromyalgia." *Scandinavian Journal of Rheumatology*. 23, no. 5 (1994): 255–259.

Yunus, M. B. et al. "A controlled study of primary fibromyalgia syndrome: clinical features and association with other functional syndromes." *Journal of Rheumatology.* 16, supple 19 (1989): 62.

Yunus, M. B. et al. "Relationship of clinical features with psychological status in primary fibromyalgia." *Arthritis Rheumatology.* 34, no. 1 (1991): 15–21.

Yunus, M. B. "The role of gender in fibromyalgia syndrome." *Curr Rheumatol Rep.* 3, no. 2 (April 2001): 128–134.

Resource Guide

American Academy of Allergy and
Immunology
611 E. Wells St.
Milwaukee, WI 53202
(414) 272-6071

American Academy of
Environmental Medicine
P.O. Box 16105
Denver, CO 80216
(303) 622-9755

American Apitherapy Society
P.O. Box 74
North Hartland, VT 05052
(802) 295-8764

American Association of
Acupuncture and Oriental
Medicine
4101 Lake Boone Tr., Ste. 201
Raleigh, NC 27607
(919) 787-5181

American Association for Chronic
Fatigue Syndrome
7 Van Buren Street
Albany, NY 12206
(518) 482-2202

American Association for Marriage
and Family Therapy
1133 15th St. NW, Ste. 300
Washington, DC 20005
(800) 374-2638

American College of
Rheumatology
60 Executive Park S., Ste. 150
Atlanta, GA 30329
(404) 633-3777

American Dietetic Association
430 N. Michigan Ave.
Chicago, IL 60611

The American Fibromyalgia
Syndrome Association, Inc.
6380 E Tanque Verde Rd. Ste. D,
Tucson, AZ 85715
(520) 733-1570

American Holistic Medical
Association
2002 Eastlake Ave. E.
Seattle, WA 98102
(206) 322-6842

American Nutritionists Association
P.O. Box 34030
Bethesda, MD 20817

American Psychiatric Association,
APA
Department AT, 1400 K St. NW
Washington DC 20005
(202) 682-6220

American Psychological
Association
750 First St. NE
Washington, DC 20002
(800) 374-3120

Ankylosing Spondylitis Association
511 N. LaCienega Blvd., Ste. 216
Los Angeles, CA 90048
(800) 777-8189
(310) 652-0609 (in California)

Arthritis Foundation
P.O. Box 19000
Atlanta, GA 30326
(800) 283-7800

The CFIDS Association of
    America, Inc.
P.O. Box 220398
Charlotte, NC 28222-0398
(800) 442-3437

Depression, Awareness,
    Recognition and Treatment
    (D/ART)
5600 Fishcers Lane, Rm. 10-85
Rockville, MD 20857
(800) 421-4211

Fibromyalgia Association of
    Central Ohio
P.O. Box 21988
Columbus OH 43221-0988
(614) 457-4222

Fibromyalgia Association of
    Greater Washington, Inc.
12210 Fairfax Towne Center, Ste.
    500
Fairfax, VA 22033
(703) 790-2324

Fibromyalgia Association of Texas
3810 Keele Dr.
Garland, TX 75041
(214) 271-5085

Fibromyalgia Educational Systems
500 Bushaway Road
Wayzata, MN 55391
(612) 473-6218 or 419-843-3153

Fibromyalgia Frontiers
P.O. Box 2373
Centreville, OH 22020
(703) 912-1727

The Fibromyalgia Network
P.O. Box 31750
Tucson, AZ 85751-1750
(800) 853-2929
fax (520) 290-5550

Fibromyalgia Times
P.O. Box 20408
Columbus, OH 43221-0990
(614) 457-4222

Food Allergy Network
4744 Holly Ave.
Fairfax, VA 22030-5647
(703) 691-3179

Inland Northwest Fibromyalgia
    Association
9209 E. Mission, Ste. B
Spokane, WA 99206
(509) 921-7741

Lupus Foundation of America
4 Research Pl., Ste. 180
Rockville, MD 20850-3226
(800) 558-0121

Massachusetts CFIDS Association
808 Main Street
Waltham, MA 02154
(617) 893-4415

National Alliance for the
Mentally Ill
200 N. Bleve Rd., Ste. 1015
Arlington, VA 22203-3754
(800) 950-6264

National Association of Social
Workers
750 First St. NE, Ste. 700
Washington, DC 20002
(202) 408-8600

National Chronic Pain Outreach
Association
7979 Old Georgetown Rd., Ste.
100
Bethesda, MD 20814
(301) 652-4948

National Commission for the
Certification of Acupuncturists
1424 16th St. NW, Ste. 501
Washington, DC 20036
(202) 232-1404

National Depressive and Manic
Depressive Association
730 N. Franklin, Ste. 501
Chicago, IL 60610
(800) 82N-DMDA or
(800) 826-3632

National Foundation for
Depressive Illness
P.O. Box 2257
New York, NY 10116
(800) 248-4344

National Institute of Arthritis and
Musculoskeletal and Skin
Diseases
NIH Information Clearinghouse

Box AMS
8000 Rockville Pike
Bethesda, MD 20892
(301) 495-4484

National Mental Health
Association
1021 Prince St.
Alexandria, VA 22314-2971
(800) 969-6642

Restless Legs Syndrome
Foundation, Inc.
304 Glenwood Ave.
Raleigh, NC 27603-1455
(919) 834-0821

Seattle Fibromyalgia International
Team, Inc.
P.O. Box 77373
Seattle, WA 98177
(206) 362-2310

The TMJ Association
6418 W. Washington Blvd.
Milwaukee, WI 53213
(414) 259-3223

Canada

Fibromyalgia Association of BC
Box 15455
Vancouver, BC V6B 5B2 Canada
(604) 430-6643

The Ontario Fibromyalgia
Association
250 Bloor Street, E. Ste. 901
Toronto, ON V4W 3P2 Canada

The Arthritis Society, BC Division
895 West 10th Avenue
Vancouver, BC V5Z 1L7 Canada
(604) 879-7511

National Institute of Arthritis and Musculoskeletal and Skin Diseases Multipurpose Centers

Boston University School
of Medicine
71 E. Concord St., K5
Boston, MA 02118
(617) 638-4310

Brigham and Women's Hospital
75 Francis St.
Boston, MA 02115
(617) 732-5356

Case Western Reserve University
2074 Abington Rd.
Cleveland, OH 44106
(216) 844-3168

Cornell University Medical College
The Hospital for Special Surgery
Research Building, Room 605
535 East 70th St.
New York, NY 10021
(212) 606-1189

Indiana Univ. School of Medicine
541 Clinical Dr., Room 492
Indianapolis, IN 46202-5103
(317) 274-4225

Northwestern University Medical
School
303 E. Chicago Ave., Ward 3-315
Chicago, IL 60611
(313) 503-8197

Stanford University
100 Welch Rd., Ste. 203
Pal Alto, CA 94304

University of Alabama at
Birmingham
UAB Station, THT 429A
Birmingham, AL 35294
(205) 934-5306

University of California, San Diego
Department of Medicine, 0945
La Jolla, CA 92093
(619) 558-1291

University of California,
San Francisco
P.O. Box 0868
San Francisco, CA 94143-0868
(415) 750-2104

University of California School
of Medicine
10833 LeConte Ave., 47-139 CHS
Los Angeles, CA 90024-1736
(213) 825-7991

University of Connecticut School
of Medicine
263 Farmington Ave.
Farmington, CT 06030-1310
(203) 679-3605

University of North Carolina at
Chapel Hill
932 FLOB, UNC-CH School of
Medicine
Chapel Hill, NC 27514
(919) 966-4191

Audio/Video and Other Materials

The Body Advantage Exercise System (1996), developed by Dr. Joe M. Elrod: A truly unique piece of exercise equipment, designed to be one of the most comprehensive and effective wellness programs available to fibromyalgics on the market today. It has a wide range of uses for people of all ages and with every level of ability or disability. Originally designed for sufferers of fibromyalgia, arthritis and other systemic conditions to help regain flexibility, this system also helps the average person seeking physical fitness by increasing flexibility and neuromuscular coordination and control. Includes resistance band, manual, video and travel pouch. For more information or to order the system, call (205) 933-5275, fax (205) 939-0368, send email to DrElrod@TheBodyAdvantage.com, or write to 1222 14th Avenue South, Suite 101, Birmingham, AL 35205.

Fibromyalgia: One-Day Seminar (1993/1994): Audiotapes of daylong forums sponsored by the Arthritis Foundation Rocky Mountain Chapter. Includes sessions by rheumatologists, neurologists, psychiatrists, psychologists, and occupational therapists. To order: Arthritis Foundation, Rock Mountain Chapter, 2280 South Albion St., Denver, CO 80222-4906, (303) 756-8622 or call (800) 475-6447 for an order blank. Website: http://www.arthritis.org. Cost: $6 each or $5 each for three or more.

What's New in Fibromyalgia? Third National Seminar (1994): Series of seven videos and 16 audiotapes about basic research, growth hormone factors, exercise, long-term outcomes, post-traumatic fibromyalgia, legal issues, coping with fibromyalgia, and a "ask the experts." Some information is too technical for the average audience, although much useful information is covered. For more information contact National Fibromyalgia Partnership, 140 Zinn Way, Linden, VA 22642, (866) 725-4404. Cost: $30 per video or $165 for a complete set of seven videos; $15 for set of two audiotapes for $75 for complete set of 13.

Aspirin and Other NSAIDs (1996): This 16-page brochure discusses aspirin and other nonsteroidal anti-inflammatory drugs, including dosage, side effects, and important tips to remember when taking them. To order one copy: Arthritis Foundation, 1330 W. Peachtree St., Atlanta, GA 30309, 800/283-7800. To order copies in multiples of 50: P.O. Box 6996, Alpharetta, GA 30329, (800) 207-8633.

Coping with Depression in A Chronic Illness (1995): This 14-page brochure is a helpful primer on coping with and accepting change. To order: Michigan Lupus Foundation, 26202 Harper Ave., St. Clair Shores, MI 48081, (810) 775-8310. Cost: $3.50 plus $1.50 shipping/handling.

The Drug Guide (1995): Originally featured in the July/ August issue of Arthritis Today, this 10-page guide will educate you about the drugs you take for your arthritis. To order one copy: Arthritis Foundation, 1330 W. Peachtree St., Atlanta, GA 30309, (800) 283-7800. To order copies in multiples of 50: P.O. Box 6996, Alpharetta, GA 30329, (800) 207-8633.

Mid-Atlantic Conference on Fibromyalgia Treatment (1996): Proceeding of the September 1996 conference are available on audiocassette. Set of six 90-minute Audiocassettes. To order: Fibromyalgia Association of Greater Washington, D.C. (FMAGW), Suite 500, 12210 Fairfax Towne Center, Fairfax, VA 22033, (703) 790-2324. Cost $72 for the general public.

The Success Journal (1996), by Dr. Joe M. Elrod. Kinner Printing/Dr. Joe M. Elrod & Associates. The Success Journal brings basic principles for successful living into a simple workable system so that you can effectively succeed in the major areas of your life. The plan is very practical and will work for you regardless of whether you are a student, an athlete, a salesperson, a manager, a housewife, a teacher, a factory worker or if you run your own business. The Success Journal helps you identify your goals and create a plan for success. In includes all the ingredients for success, including planning charts, helpful information and inspirational tips. For mor information or to order, call (334) 272-3605 or write to 3066 Zelda Road, Suite 212, Montgomery, AL 36106.

The Fibromyalgia Nutrition Guide, by Mary Moeller, L.P.N., and Dr. Joe M. Elrod. Contains valuable dietary guidelines, 150 recipes and more for overcoming fibromyalgia, chronic fatigue syndrome, migraines, sleep disorders and other chronic conditions.

The Body Advantage Newsletter, by The HOPE Medical Clinic and Dr. Joe M. Elrod. The newsletter is published quarterly and contains the latest research on new treatments, medications, natural supplements, nutrition, exercise, stress, pain and sleep. Also contains success stories, articles, and answers to most common questions. Subscriptions are available. Use phone, fax, address or email information below to order.

To contact Dr. Elrod regarding consultation, speaking engagements, or for other information, use the following:

Dr. Joe M. Elrod
P.O. Box 43542
Birmingham, AL 35242
phone: (205) 933-5275
fax: (205) 969-8140
email: DrElrod@TheBodyAdvantage.com
website: http://www.TheBodyAdvantage.com

Index

About the Author

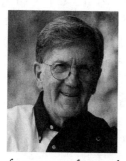 Dr. Elrod holds multiple degrees in exercise physiology and has completed post-doctoral research in the areas of nutrition, exercise physiology, heart disease, cancer and arthritis. A former professor, he is now a health consultant who has worked with various groups, including AT&T, McDonalds, NASA and various university medical student organizations.

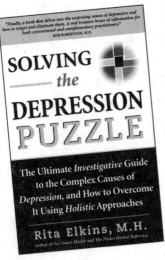
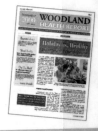